CHEMICAL ENGINEERING METHODS AND TECHNOLOGY

CYANIDE

OCCURRENCE, CHARACTERISTICS AND APPLICATIONS

CHEMICAL ENGINEERING METHODS AND TECHNOLOGY

Additional books in this series can be found on Nova's website under the Series tab.

Additional e-books in this series can be found on Nova's website under the e-book tab.

ENVIRONMENTAL SCIENCE, ENGINEERING AND TECHNOLOGY

Additional books in this series can be found on Nova's website under the Series tab.

Additional e-books in this series can be found on Nova's website under the e-book tab.

CHEMICAL ENGINEERING METHODS AND TECHNOLOGY

CYANIDE

OCCURRENCE, CHARACTERISTICS AND APPLICATIONS

BENITO SOTO-BLANCO
EDITOR

NOVINKA

New York

For permission to use material from this book please contact us:
Telephone 631-231-7269; Fax 631-231-8175
Web Site: http://www.novapublishers.com

Library of Congress Cataloging-in-Publication Data

ISBN: 978-1-62618-297-4

Published by Nova Science Publishers, Inc. † New York

Contents

Preface		**vii**
Chapter 1	The Role of Hydrogen Cyanide in the Origin of Life *Alicia Negrón-Mendoza, Alejandro Heredia, Maria Colín-García and Sergio Ramos Bernal*	**1**
Chapter 2	Cyanide Poisoning in Animals and Humans *Antônio Carlos Lopes Câmara and Benito Soto-Blanco*	**23**
Chapter 3	Estimating the Hydrogen Cyanide Generation: Thermodynamics and Mass Transfer *Humberto Estay*	**47**
Chapter 4	Application of Cyanide-Bridged Coordination Polymers for Electrode Materials of Rechargeable Batteries *Masashi Okubo*	**87**
Index		**111**

PREFACE

Cyanide is a omnipresent substance in the environment and might participated in the chemical evolution processes before the appearance of life on Earth. Now-a-days this compound is released by several processes, including acrylic and ammonia manufacturing,electroplating, steel production, the extraction of gold and silver,and jewelry. Hydrocyanic acid is also found in smoke, and it is generated by the incomplete combustion of carbon compounds in fires, cigarettes and propulsion motors. Furthermore, over 2,500 plant species are known to accumulate cyanide. In this book, the authors present several aspects of cyanide. In the first chapter, the role of cyanide in the chemical evolution process on early Earth and beyond our planet. The toxicity of cyanide to animals and humans are presented at chapter 2.In the third chapter, the authorpurposesa phenomenological method to estimate the hydrogen cyanide generation.The last chapter is a review of use the cyanide-bridged coordination polymer electrodes in electrode materials of rechargeable batteries.

Chapter 1 - "The role of hydrogen cyanide in the origin of life", by Alicia Negrón-Mendoza, Alejandro Heredia, Maria Colín-García, and Sergio Ramos Bernal - Chemical evolution encompasses physical and chemical processes that took place on Earth before the appearance of life. To simulate the chemical process that may have occurred, a heterogeneous medium is geologically more likely to succeed than a homogeneous phase. The main interest of this research is to stress the relevance of radiation chemistry as a tool to elucidate the importance of ionizing radiation to study the formation of biologically-relevant compounds from HCN and its derivatives and to remark on the importance of the chemical reactions that may occur at hydrosphere/lithosphere interfaces. To this end, the authors study the adsorption capacity of HCN in different surface minerals that may have been present in the primordial epoch and study the chemical reactions that occur when the system HCN-mineral surface is exposed to a high-energy source. These studies show that HCN can be adsorbed readily from the surfaces studied. This adsorption is influenced by pH and type of adsorbent. Irradiation of HCN solutions produced simple organic compounds and an oligomeric material that, upon hydrolysis, yields compounds of biological importance such as amino acids, carboxylic acids, and purines. These products are formed even at low temperatures and low radiation doses. This work strongly reinforces the hypothesis of the central role of HCN as a parent molecule in the process of chemical evolution on early Earth, comets, and other extraterrestrial environments and the use of ionizing radiation as an energy source to induce chemical changes in these systems.

Chapter 2 - “Cyanide poisoning in animals and humans” , by Benito Soto-Blanco and Antônio Carlos Lopes Câmara - Cyanide is a ubiquitous substance in the environment. It can be released from cyanogenic plants, industrial processes (such as metal processing, electroplating, and acrylic and chemical synthesis), and medicinal drugs (such as nitroprusside). Cyanide inhibits several cellular enzymes, including cytochrome oxidase, which is a key enzyme in the cellular respiratory chain. Most of the cyanide absorbed by an organism is detoxified by enzymatic combination with sulfur, and acute poisoning occurs when detoxification systems are overwhelmed. Acute cyanide poisoning is potentially fatal and is a result of cellular hypoxia and cytotoxic anoxia. Long-term exposure to cyanide is responsible for various toxic effects, including reduced weight gain, damage to the liver, impaired thyroid function, and neuropathies. Furthermore, various experimental studies and field cases in several animal species have verified that exposure to cyanide or to cyanogenic plants results in reproductive disturbances.

Chapter 3 - “Estimating the hydrogen cyanide generation: thermodynamic and mass transfer”, by Humberto Estay - The industries related to the production or use of cyanide must ensure high safety standards in order to minimize the risk to personnel exposed to hydrogen cyanide (HCN). This can be reached by accomplishing a global search of all parameters involved in the process, taking also into account the local regulations for HCN emanations. In this scenario, there is a high interest in developing methods capable of quantifying the HCN generation in different processes or equipments and in that way the implementation of remediation actions in the process operations or in the design of future projects can be taken. Nowadays, the most used method to estimate HCN generation is based on the dissociation curve of free cyanide and the Henry's law constant. However, this method overestimates consistently the volatilized HCN in the exit gases due to there is no inclusion of the chemical interactions of cyanide with others species (e.g., zinc, copper, and nickel), and neither considers the mass transfer of HCN, the most influential factor in the volatilization of HCN. The mass transfer of HCN in the liquid phase represents the main resistance of HCN transport into the gas phase, which is dependent on the characteristics of the system such as geometry, hydrodynamic and state conditions. With this background in mind, a phenomenological method to estimate the HCN generation in any system is proposed. This theoretical method is mainly based on the thermodynamic equilibrium of the different cyanide complex species present in a solution, the phase equilibrium behaviour based on the Henry's law equilibrium, and the mass transfer of HCN into the air based on a resistances-in-series model to determine the HCN content in the liquid and gas phases. In addition, the proposed method also evaluates the effect of system conditions (such as temperature, pressure and pH) and the characteristics of the operation or equipment used. Thus, this phenomenological method can be a powerful and valuable tool for quantifying of HCN generation in realistic simulations, along with providing rapid identification of risk conditions in the process and more alternatives for investment project decision making.

Chapter 4 - "Application of cyanide-bridged coordination polymers for electrode materials of rechargeable batteries", by Masashi Okubo - Development of novel host materials with enhanced ion storage ability is of particular importance in a wide range of applications, especially the electrode materials for batteries. A cyanide-bridged coordination polymer is one of the most attractive host materials, because both the ionic-diffusion channel and electron conduction path frequently coexist within the framework. For example, a cyanide-bridged perovskite-type framework, so-called Prussian blue analog (PBA), has been studied intensively for decades from the viewpoint of electrochromism. However, the electrochemical properties, *i.e.*, electrochemical ion intercalation/extraction of PBAs can also be applied to the electrode materials of the batteries. In this chapter, the solid state electrochemistry of PBA is briefly explained. Then, the cyanide-bridged coordination polymer electrodes for the battery application are reviewed.

In: Cyanide
Editor: Benito Soto-Blanco
ISBN: 978-1-62618-297-4

Chapter 1

THE ROLE OF HYDROGEN CYANIDE IN THE ORIGIN OF LIFE

Alicia Negrón-Mendoza[1], Alejandro Heredia[1], Maria Colín-García[2] and Sergio Ramos Bernal[1]
[1]Instituto de Ciencias Nucleares,
Universidad Nacional Autónoma de México
[2]Instituto de Geología,
Universidad Nacional Autónoma de México, México, Mexico

ABSTRACT

Chemical evolution encompasses physical and chemical processes that took place on Earth before the appearance of life. To simulate the chemical process that may have occurred, a heterogeneous medium is geologically more likely to succeed than a homogeneous phase. The main interest of this research is to stress the relevance of radiation chemistry as a tool to elucidate the importance of ionizing radiation to study the formation of biologically-relevant compounds from HCN and its derivatives and to remark on the importance of the chemical reactions that may occur at hydrosphere/lithosphere interfaces. To this end, we study the adsorption capacity of HCN in different surface minerals that may have been present in the primordial epoch and study the chemical reactions that occur when the system HCN-mineral surface is exposed to a high-energy source. These studies show that HCN can be adsorbed readily from the surfaces studied. This adsorption is influenced by pH and type of adsorbent. Irradiation of HCN solutions produced simple organic compounds and an oligomeric material that, upon hydrolysis, yields compounds of biological importance such as amino acids, carboxylic acids, and purines. These products are formed even at low temperatures and low radiation doses. This work strongly reinforces the hypothesis of the central role of HCN as a parent molecule in the process of chemical evolution on early Earth, comets, and other extraterrestrial environments and the use of ionizing radiation as an energy source to induce chemical changes in these systems.

1. Introduction

1.1. What is Chemical Evolution?

The Oparin-Haldane hypothesis states that life originated via the abiotic synthesis and subsequent accumulation of organic compounds, through a series of physical and chemical processes, collectively known as chemical evolution. In a more practical sense, chemical evolution is the chemistry of the formation and organization of bio-organic compounds under conditions that are assumed to be geologically and astronomically primitive (Negrón-Mendoza and Albarrán, 1993).

Although chemical evolution is a perfectly defined process, it cannot be precisely defined spatially or temporally. However, it was likely due to the Earth's surface becoming hospitable enough after it cooled to allow the synthesis of organic molecules (Draganić et al., 1978) and decreased when the first living system emerged. Both events are difficult to identify conclusively because of a lack of techniques or because the record was destroyed by the planet's own geophysical processes.

The processes of chemical evolution were not exclusive to Earth. The same type of reactions that gave rise to the biologically important compounds on our planet may occur elsewhere in the Solar System, such as comets, meteorites, interstellar dust grains, or even other planets or their satellites. Terrestrial planets have a solid silicate surface as a key component, which could actively participate in chemical evolution events. This surface is made up of different types of minerals that are indicative of geological events.

1.2. When Did Chemical Evolution Accomplish?

The Solar System originated 4500 or 4600 million years ago (Could, 1977; Trimble, 1997), while the oldest fossil record indicates that life existed as such for about 3300-3500 million years ago (Schopf and Packer, 1987). This leaves a few million years (in a geological scale) for life to evolve from the so called primordial soup to an RNA world and finally to the DNA and protein system. Oparin and Haldane suggested that the process took several million years to develop. However, Lazcano-Araujo and Miller (1994) proposed that the chemical reactions probably occurred quickly. They propose that the origin and early evolution of life would not have taken much more than 10 million years.

1.3. Available Energy Sources for the Processes of Chemical Evolution

To synthesize organic molecules, a source of energy was needed to induce the chemical changes in the raw material. Different energy sources have been proposed to contribute to organic synthesis. In this section, we review the energy sources available on the early Earth and on extraterrestrial bodies, for example, those that should be important in altering the nature of comets in outer space (Negrón-Mendoza and Albarrán, 1993).

1.3.1. Energy Sources in the Early Earth

The following energy sources are typically considered viable on early Earth: the sonic energy caused by the impacts of objects; cosmic rays, which should have represented a good source of energy; the thermal energy generated by volcanoes, which was able to promote the synthesis of organic compounds by pyrolysis; the UV radiation emitted by the Sun, which is by far considered the most important source of energy due to its ability to generate photolytic reactions in the upper atmosphere; and finally, radioactivity, the main action of which was in the lithosphere.

1.3.2. Ionizing Radiation as an Energy Source in Chemical Evolution

The use of ionizing radiation as an energy source stems from the calculation of the decay of radioactive elements such as ^{40}K, ^{235}U, ^{238}U, and ^{232}Th, all of which have half-lives in the order of 10^9 years or more. Several other naturally radioactive isotopes with long half-lives have been discovered, such as ^{87}Rb, ^{115}Y, and ^{138}La, and could have been important in prebiotic time. A large number of short-lived radioactive isotopes may have contributed to the prebiotic synthesis in the early history of the Earth. However, all isotopes with a half-life in the order of 10^9 years or less have since been reduced to immeasurable small fractions of their original amounts (Birch, 1954). Under the present conditions of the Earth, the irradiation effects of these radionuclides are quite negligible. Nonetheless, those isotopes may have been very important in prebiotic synthesis.

Ionizing radiation energy is important for the following reasons: it has a specific energy deposition (this means the energy is deposited over a distance of penetration); the effect is independent of the temperature or concentration of solutions; its efficiency in producing free radicals; and it promotes chemical processes, even in the hostile conditions of prebiotic chemistry, like those in the ocean depths, the underground waters of primitive Earth, or in comets and matter in space (Draganić, 2000). In addition, it is able to induce chemical reactions in different aggregation states. The main contribution of ionizing radiation is due to its efficiency in inducing chemical reactions, its abundance, and its wide distribution.

Sources of ionizing radiation can be terrestrial or extraterrestrial. Extraterrestrial ionizing radiation includes cosmic rays and UV radiation, while internal sources are due to the radionuclides present in the planet.

1.3.3. Radioactive Element Distribution on the Earth

The distribution of radioisotopes is largely determined by geophysical conditions that existed in various stages of Earth development. Although ^{40}K, ^{96}Zr, ^{43}Ca, and ^{232}Th are the most widespread isotopes in the Earth's crust, ^{40}K is by far the most important of these radionuclides since it is evenly distributed in the terrestrial crust, especially in persilicic magmatic rocks, in clays, shells, and in the ocean. The presence of radionuclides in oceans, lakes, and ponds is an important factor because these elements were able to react freely in an ionized form. Those dissolved ions produced an environment in which simple organic compounds could have been synthesized or modified.

In the case of Earth's crust, it is possible to calculate the corresponding amount of energy available at 4550 million years ago in the form of ionizing radiation and heat (from the rates at which the major long-lived radioactive species, ^{40}K, ^{235}U, ^{238}U, ^{232}Th, decay). The amount of radioactivity per unit of time has dropped three to four times the present value. Mosqueira et al. (1996) have estimated the annual dose (in Gy/year) at 3800 million years ago (a probable origin of life) in sites of interest to prebiotic chemistry, such as clays, sedimentary rocks, or the oceans.

The localized nature of radiation from other radionuclides, like uranium or thorium, may have produced microenvironments of high activity, in which simple organics could be condensed into more complex molecules. In fact, mineral deposits associated with these radioisotopes may have shown catalytic activity. In this regard, the important role that clay and clay minerals played in chemical evolution has been recognized (Bernal, 1951). Clay minerals are selectively efficient in fixing potassium; one consequence of this fixation is the highest value of radioactivity found in clays (see Table I). This amount is estimated at 25×10^9 Ci per kg (21×10^9 Ci per kg is due to ^{40}K, and 1.4×10^9 Ci per kg to ^{235}U). In our research, both radiation and catalyses have been experimentally tested to evaluate their contribution to chemical evolution processes (Negrón-Mendoza et al., 2010).

1.3.4. Ionizing Radiation Contribution in Extraterrestrial Environments

A great number of molecules have been detected in interstellar space and other bodies of the Solar System. The importance of energy sources and their distribution in interstellar space is of primary interest because they are the responsible for the formation of complex organics in space, including environments like interstellar molecular clouds, comets, asteroids, and interplanetary dust particles. These energy sources include cosmic rays, a flux of ubiquitous particles (protons, helium nuclei, and the nuclei of heavy elements), solar wind, gamma rays, and magnetospheric particles (Stern, 2003).

Table I. Estimated annual dose (Gy/year at 3800 million years ago at the Earth´s crust§).

Material	^{40}K	^{238}U	^{232}Th
Sedimentary rock (total)	2.74×10^{-2}	3×10^{-3}	1.52×10^{-3}
Igneous rocks (total)	5.2×10^{-2}	3.3×10^{-3}	4.2×10^{-3}
Deep sea sediments			
Clays	1.75×10^{-2}	6.1×10^{-4}	6.9×10^{-4}
Carbonates	2×10^{-3}		
Seawater	2.5×10^{-4}	1.42×10^{-6}	1.98×10^{-9}

§Modified from Mosqueira et al., 1996. Gy=gray, Gray is the metric measurementunit (SI) of absorbed radiation dose of ionizing radiation=1 J/kg) of matter.

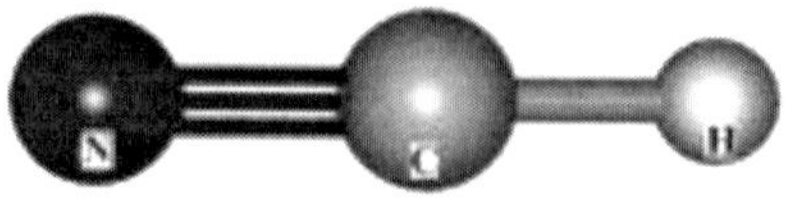

Figure 1. Hydrogen cyanide molecule showing its triple bond C≡N and linear molecule.

2. HYDROGEN CYANIDE (HCN)

Hydrogen cyanide, a very simple molecule, played an important role in chemical evolution processes due to its unique physical and chemical properties. It weights 27.03 g/mol, and its boiling and melting points are low (26 °C and –13 °C, respectively). It is less dense than water (approximately one third), but highly miscible in water. Chemically, it is a very reactive molecule due its triple bond C≡N (see Figure 1).

2.1. Biologically Occurring HCN Derivatives

Despite its toxicity, HCN is widely distributed in biological nature. Many organisms exhibit the phenomenon of cyanogenesis or are able to metabolize this compound. Among them, some plants (Nartey, 1981), bacteria (Castric, 1981), fungi (Fry and Myers, 1981), and a very specific group of animals, arthropods, exhibit cyanogenesis (Duffey, 1981).

In plants, the ability to free HCN depends on the rate of synthesis and the accumulation capacity. HCN can accumulate on leaves, stems, fruits, seeds, roots, and tubers. In plants, cyanogenic material is located in the vacuoles, while hydrolytic enzymes are cytoplasmic (Nartey, 1981). There is a direct relationship between plants' resistance to pathogenic fungi and their ability to metabolize HCN. In the latter, tolerance was found to be induced by HCN (Fry and Evans, 1977), as if it were a coevolutionary process. Many fungi are capable of incorporating hydrogen cyanide in amino acids such as alanine, asparagine, and glutamic acid (Fry and Mayers, 1981). Bacteria are capable of synthesizing HCN to metabolize by two major pathways, β–cyanoalanine and cyano acid-β–γ-aminobutyric acid (Castric, 1981).

2.2. HCN as a Key Molecule in Chemical Evolution Studies

An interesting question connected to chemical evolution is the extent to which the basic building blocks of life can be synthesized on the Earth, as well as in the interstellar medium from simple molecules like HCN. The detection of amino acids and other complex organic compounds in meteorites and comets implies that the formation of molecules, some of them of biological importance, is possible. This finding opens the possibility that these bodies may contribute to the inventory of organic molecules on the early Earth.

Table II. Formation of Biologically Important Compounds from HCN and its derivatives.

Reagents ,	Conditions	Products	References
HCN	In basic aqueous solution	Adenine	Oró and Kimball, 1961.
HCN	Basic solution. UV radiation	Adenine, guanine	Ponnamperuma and Mack, 1965.
HCN	Milder basic conditions	Diaminomalonitrile	Ferris and Orgel, 1966.
Thermal HCN oligomers	Acid hydrolysis	Purines, pyrimidines, on hydrolysis yields amino acids	Matthews and Moser, 1966.
HCN	Gamma radiolysis of aqueous solution at pH 6	Purines, pyrimidines, on hydrolysis yields amino acids, carboxylic acids	Draganić et al., 1984a, 1984b.
Radiation-induced HCN oligomers	Hydrolysis in mild conditions	Purines, pyrimidines, amino acids, carboxylic acids	Negrón-Mendoza and Draganić, 1984. Colín-García et al., 2009.
Cyanamide	Basic solution	Guanine	Levy et al., 1999.
Cyanamide	Basic solutions	Ala, leu, phe peptides	Hawker Jr and Oró, 1981.
HCN	Gamma radiolysis of adsorbed HCN in clays	Purines, pyrimidines, on hydrolysis amino acids, carboxylic acids	Colín-García et al., 2009.
HCN	Low temperature	Adenine, guanine, glycine	Levy et al., 1999; 2000.
Cyanamide	Gamma radiolysis at pH 2 and 5	Urea, biuret, arginine, methylamine-azoformamida	Draganić et al., 1978.
RCN	Gamma radiation in solution	Carboxylic acids, amino acids	Draganić et al., 1973.

HCN, and its derivatives, are among the most widely distributed molecules in the interstellar medium (Irvine, 1998; Boonman et al., 2001). The occurrence and formation of HCN came from several sources, both terrestrial (e.g., volcanic eruptions) and extraterrestrial (e.g., comets and interstellar space). Hydrogen cyanide has been observed in volcanic emissions (Mukhin, 1974). Nitriles are especially important in extraterrestrial environments. Methane-nitrogen-rich atmospheres, like that of Titan, contain HCN, C_2N_2 and HC_3N (Vuitton et al., 2006). CN, CN^+, HCN, and CH_3CN have been found in comets. Nitriles have been detected in circumstellar envelopes (Matthews and Sears, 1986) and dark clouds (Johansson et al., 1984). They have also been discovered in the atmospheres of some stars, in satellites, and the tail of comets (Ip et al., 1990; Magee-Sauer et al., 1999). In those bodies, the HCN molecule is one of the most important reagents. Equally important is the same HCN or its polymers may have played critical roles in the irradiation process of ices, both cometary and those of the ISM (Gerakines et al., 2004).

In 1924, when A. I. Oparin proposed the theory of the origin of life, CN and HCN had been detected in the Solar System, particularly in the spectra of comets. In fact, this was one of the fundamental reasons for Oparin's assertion that chemical evolution was the preamble to the emergence of life on Earth (Oró et al., 1982).

2.3. Synthesis of HCN in Prebiotic Conditions

Many of the compounds essential to life can be synthesized from simple molecules; key molecules include hydrogen cyanide (HCN) and CN-containing molecules. They are abundantly formed in various gas mixtures of simple compounds using different energy sources such as UV light (Toupance et al., 1978) and electric discharges (Chada et al., 1971). The formation of HCN in simulated Jovian atmospheric experiments was demonstrated by Woeller and Ponnamperuma (1969); it also formed during Gupta et al.'s simulation of the atmosphere of Titan in 1981. The synthesis of HCN and other nitriles from a mixture of CO, NH_3, and H_2 in a Fisher Tropsch reaction was carried out by Anderson in 1984. The photolysis of CH_4 and NH_3 produced HCN (Ferris and Chen, 1975). There are numerous other scenarios that also established the formation of HCN and other simple nitriles.

Thermal polymers of HCN were described earlier in the literature and their importance has been shown; much effort has been paid elucidating the structure of the HCN polymer (Matthews and Minard, 2008). Joan Oró (Oró et al., 1982) suggested that HCN was one of the key compounds in the synthesis of biochemical compounds needed for the emergence of life due to its reactivity and ability to condense with itself and with other compounds. Moreover, HCN has shown its ample role as a precursor to bio-molecules in chemical evolution experiments in which various energy sources were used.

HCN is a volatile molecule (b.p. 26 °C) and polymerization may not occur in environments where its concentration was very low in the early Earth, so the concentration mechanisms should have been fundamental. Many mechanisms have been proposed for concentration, but the most important are those that involve the participation of solid surfaces. The role of solid surfaces could include several mechanisms, such as adsorption or freezing, which implies the intervention of minerals (such as clays, Figure 2) or the formation of ice (Miller and Orgel, 1974).

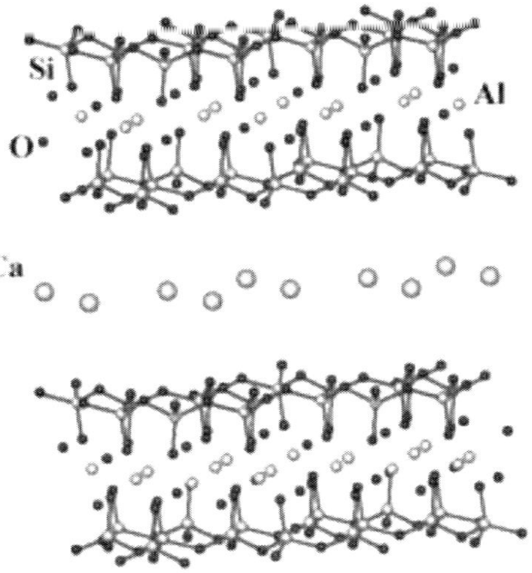

Figure 2. Calcium montmorillonite has a very high surface/area ratio and consequently exposes different chemical groups.

The polymerization of HCN is a spontaneous and exothermic process that forms HCN polymers in a wide variety of conditions initiated by bases such ammonia or free radicals from ionizing radiation and occurs in a wide range of temperatures and pressures in both polar (H_2O) or non polar (hydrocarbons) phases (Matthews and Minard, 2008). Thermal polymers were described very early in the literature (Negrón-Mendoza and Ramos-Bernal, 1998 and the references therein). Much effort has been made to elucidate their structure. HCN polymers released upon hydrolysis a measurable quantity of amino acids and nucleic acid bases, the building blocks of proteins and nucleic acid, respectively.

There have been many studies showing how small molecules such as HCN, ammonia, and simple aldehydes can be converted into prebiotic monomers like amino acids. The famous experiment performed by Miller (1953), in which an electric discharge in a mixture of methane, ammonia, water, and hydrogen produced several amino acids and carboxylic acids, is explained via the Strecker synthesis by the *in situ* synthesis of HCN.

2.4. HCN and RCN Radiolysis

2.4.1. Homogeneous Phase

Radiation-induced reactions have been proposed as a mechanism for synthesizing organic compounds under conditions that presumably existed when life on Earth began. Simple precursors cause a large variety of compounds in radiation-induced reactions. Free radical processes that are initiated by ionizing radiation in aqueous solutions of various simple cyano-containing compounds lead to the formation of a large number of compounds of interest in chemical evolution studies. Several dozen short-lived intermediates have been identified; the rate constants of the reactions were determined, and using the free radical model of water radiolysis, a reasonable insight into the observed process can often be achieved. Of particular interest in the studies in chemical evolution is that these radiation-induced changes can take place under a large range of conditions—pH, temperature, absorbed dose, solute concentration, the presence of other chemical compounds, etc. (Draganić et al., 1984b, Negrón-Mendoza and Draganić, 1984).

Radiation chemistry deals with chemical changes induced by ionizing radiation. Knowledge of the chemical effects produced by high-energy radiation is sufficiently well founded. The principal characteristic of high-energy radiation is that it causes excitation and ionization in all materials. Many of the principles of radiation chemistry are applied to liquid phases and have been developed in the course of studies on chemical evolution and water solutions. The radiolysis of water and aqueous solutions has been studied because of the role they play in chemistry, including chemical evolution.

Interaction with radiation depends on electron density; therefore, a substance with a low atomic number as a minor component of a mixture (a solute in aqueous solution for example) will only absorb a small proportion of the radiation. Radiation acts directly on the major component (direct effect), forming radicals and other chemical species. These reactive species may react with the minor component to yield products (an indirect effect). These products are the most important in aqueous solutions. Although, there is much energy involved in the radiation—many times the energy needed to break chemical bonds—the species produced are identifiable chemical species and undergo chemical reactions according to consistent, established mechanisms (Spinks and Woods, 1990).

The passage of high-energy radiation through water or dilute aqueous solutions (represented by ww——>) initially yields electrons, positively-charged water ions, and excited water molecules, which are represented by an asterisk (*):

H_2O ww——> $H_3O^+ + e^-$

H_2O ww——> H_2O^*

These species, through a complex mechanism, give rise to the radiolytic products of water decomposition, namely, molecular products (H_2 and H_2O_2) and radical products ($^{\cdot}H$, $^{\cdot}OH$ and e_{aq}^-). They are called primary species and are formed in a fix yield at the same conditions. The overall chemical action of radiation on water can summarized as follows:

H_2O ww——> H_2, H_2O_2, $^{\cdot}H$, $^{\cdot}OH$, e_{aq}^-

Radiolytic products are located near radiation pathways and diffuse away from reacting among themselves or with the solute present in water. Generally, the rates of these reactions are in the order of 10^5 to 10^9. These types of reactions are called diffuse control reactions.

The radiolytic behaviors of some nitriles and cyanides in aqueous solutions in an oxygen-free atmosphere have been systematically studied (Draganić et al., 1973). Hydrogen cyanide and simple nitriles are very reactive molecules. The main attack by the water radiolytic products is in the triple bond C≡N and independent of the substituent. Fast kinetic techniques as pulse radiolysis and competition kinetics have been very successful in understanding the reaction mechanism and evaluating the rate constant. The additional reaction to the triple bond is more important, although other reactions also take part. The behavior under irradiation of RCN compounds depend on the nature of R due to its inductive and mesomeric effects. Also, the pH of the solution has consequences in the yield of the decomposition of the solute, especially in cyanides (Draganić et al., 1973). The intermediaries produced in these systems are disproportionate, dimerized, and able to give rise to a large variety of final products. About thirty radiolytic products have been identified. In a diluted solution and at low doses (in the kGy region), about 50-80 % of the C and N atoms of the decomposed RCN molecules form more complex molecules, mainly oligomers (as polyamides and polyesters). Figure 3 shows the formation of the oligomers via the irradiation of HCN solutions.

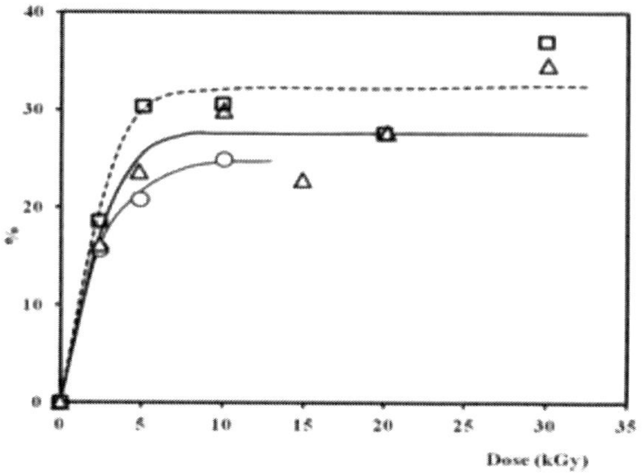

Figure 3. Effect of the irradiation dose in the formation of the oligomer (16,000 Da), at different concentrations of HCN: Legend: (o) 1×10^{-3} M; (Δ) 5×10^{-3}M; (□) 10×10^{-3} M.

Among the products detected in HCN and other simple nitriles are gaseous products such as hydrogen, carbon dioxide, carbon monoxide, methane, and ammonia. Other products are aldehydes and ketones, carboxylic acids, urea, amino acids, diaminomalonitrile, and nucleo-bases such as adenine. Figure 4 shows a gas chromatogram of the acids formed from HCN solutions after hydrolysis of the oligomeric product. The release of amino acids on hydrolysis and the positive Biuret reaction suggest the presence of peptide-type material in irradiated samples. The molecular weights of the oligomeric products are up to 20,000 Daltons throughout the dose range studied. Their amounts gradually change with increasing doses above 300 kGy: The compounds with MW between 2,000 and 6,000 Daltons become more abundant, while the amounts of polymers with MW between 6,000 and 20,000 decreases.

2.4.2. Heterogeneous Phase

To simulate chemical processes that may occur in the primitive Earth, a heterogeneous medium is geologically more likely than a homogeneous phase. For this reason, many experiments have been focused on investigating the role of mineral surfaces in prebiotic processes. In many of the proposed environments, solid surfaces are involved in the synthesis, concentration, selection, and organization of bio-molecules. The processes involved three main factors: (a) an increase in the concentration of reactants, (b) the catalysis of some reactions, and (c) the protection of products against destructive energy sources. In this way, mineral surfaces may have facilitated a transition from geochemistry to biochemistry. Among the most important solid mineral surfaces are those characterized by silicates, such as olivine, which is one of the most abundant minerals on Earth, as well as carbonates, sulfides, and clays. Environments that include olivine-rich mafic and ultramafic rocks are susceptible to chemical weathering by dissolution and hydrolysis, primarily giving rise to serpentine and magnetite.

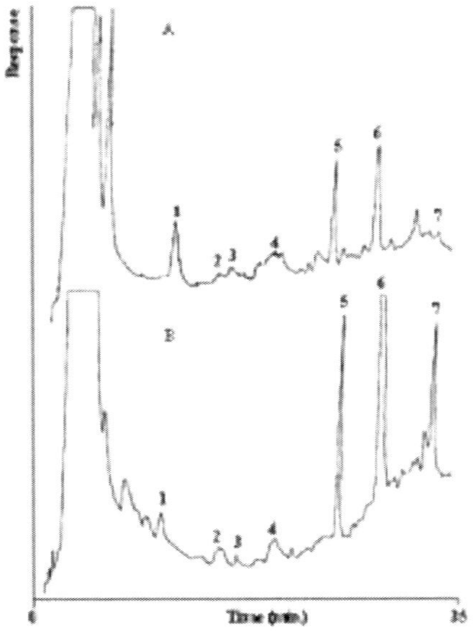

Figure 4. Gas chromatogram of the acids (as their methyl esters) formed from the radiolysis of 0.15 M oxygen-free solution of HCN. A) Irradiated at 293 K with a dose of 672 kGy and B) irradiated at 77 K at 37.5 kGy. Legend: 1. Oxalic acid, 2. Malonic acid, 3. Succinic acid, 4. Glutaric acid, 5. Carboxysuccinic acid, 6. Tricarballylic acid, and 7. Citric acid.

Table III. A summary of the general reaction scheme for the radiolysis of hydrogen cyanide.

	Reaction	k at 25 °C
	H_2O ww—> OH, H, e_{aq}^-, H_2, H_2O_2	
	Reactions with OH	
1	HCN + OH $\rightarrow$ HC(OH)=N or HC=NOH)	$k_1 = 6 \times 10^7\ M^{-1}sec^{-1}$
2	HCN + H $\rightarrow$ HC(H)=N (or HC=NH)	$k_2 = 7 \times 10^9\ M^{-1}sec^{-1}$
3	HCN + H $\rightarrow$ HC(H)=N (or HC=NH)	$k_3 = 4 \times 10^7\ M^{-1}sec^{-1}$
	Reactions with H	
4	HCN + H $\rightarrow$ HC(H)=N (or HC=NH)	$k_4 = 3.6 \times 10^7\ M^{-1}sec^{-1}$
	Reactions with e_{aq}^-	
5	HCN + H $\rightarrow$ HC(H)=N (or HC=NH)	$k_5 = 6.6 \times 10^7\ M^{-1}sec^{-1}$
6	$HCN)^-$ + H_2O $\rightarrow$ HC(H)=N (or HC=NH) + OH	k_6 very fast
7	$2H_2C$=N (or 2HC=NH) $\rightarrow$ HCN (+ H_2 $\rightarrow$ HCH=O + NH_3)	
8	NH_2C=O + NH_2 $\rightarrow$ $NH_2C(=O)NH_2$ (urea)	
9	H_2C=N (or HC=NH) + n HCN (or ^-CN) $\rightarrow$ oligomers	
10	HC(OH)=N (or HC=NOH) + nHCN or (^-CN) $\rightarrow$ oligomers	

To this end, it is necessary to study the adsorption capacity of HCN in a different mineral surface that may have been present in terrestrial and extraterrestrial environments during the primordial epoch. Second, studying the chemical reactions induced by the irradiation of HCN that occurs when the system HCN-surface is exposed to a high-energy source is also important.

Minerals' role is fundamental from this perspective because they could have behaved as concentration agents, catalysts, or shields. The exact details for those reactions and interactions are not fully known.

2.4.2. Absorption Processes

Adsorption experiments indicate that there is indeed an interaction between the HCN molecule and all of the proven minerals. HCN is highly adsorbed on all the surfaces studied, and the adsorption is pH-dependent as minerals might be activated by acids (Steudel et al., 2009) alteration of non-swelling clay minerals.

The mineral presenting with greater adsorption is dolomite, followed by zeolite and serpentine, while the mineral with a lower adsorption is olivine. It is necessary to evaluate the retention of adsorbate molecules on the surface of the adsorbent and know if adsorption is generated by a chemical interaction, or physical. These preliminary experiments show that the surfaces have a different capacity, which depends on the nature of the adsorbed. One of the most important features is the porosity. For example, dolomite (which is a calcium and magnesium carbonate) is one of the most important components of petroleum reservoir rocks. Dolomite (rocks formed by this mineral) becomes very porous in acidic solutions, which explains why HCN adsorbs on it. Zeolite, on the other hand, presents with a high adsorption rate due to the presence of specific channels in its structure; hydrogen cyanide is a small molecule and can thus easily penetrate zeolite. Olivine, however, which has no channels and is very dense, retains HCN to a lesser extent.

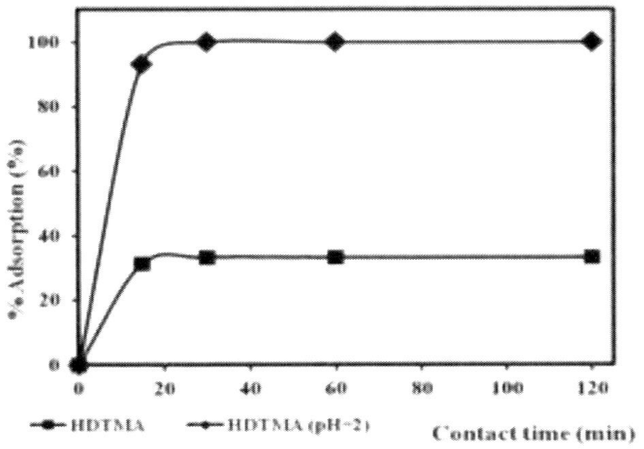

Figure 5 . Adsorption of HCN in Na^{+}-montmorillonite at pH 2, with the interlamellar channel free (♦) and (■) blocked with HDTMA.

The percentage of adsorption of sodium montmorillonite was 58% at pH 6. This percentage increased at pH 2, and the HCN is fully adsorbed by the clay (Fig. 5). However, when the clay is blocked in the interlamellar channel with quaternary ammonium salt (bromide of hexadecyl trimethyl ammonium, HDTMA), the percentage of adsorption is reduced to 33% (Figure. 5). This implies that the adsorption of HCN in this clay takes place at the interlamellar channel.

2.4.3. Radiolysis in Heterogeneous Phase

For a first approach into the radiation chemistry of HCN, the behavior under irradiation of this compound was studied in the presence of olivine, a widely distributed mineral in extraterrestrial bodies such as meteorites and comets, and serpentine -a weathering product of olivine. The results show that the presence of olivine accelerates decomposition behavior, but the presence of serpentine does not affect the decomposition rate.

The interaction of ionizing radiation with solids produces both excitation and degradation. However, storage and transfer of energy from the solid to the molecule that it is interacting with also occurs. The rate of HCN decomposition by gamma irradiation was found to be enhanced in the presence of the solid (Figure 6).

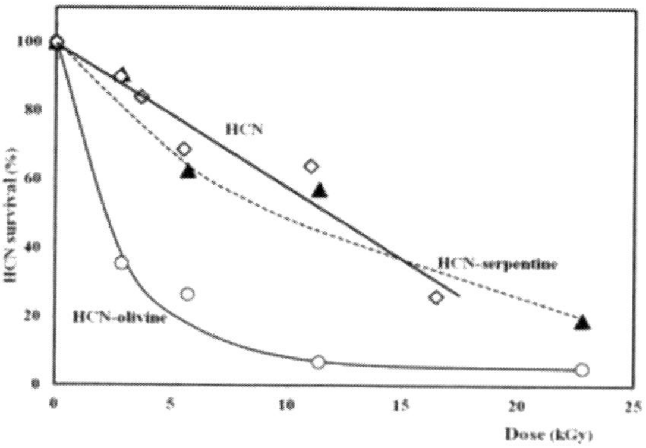

Figure 6. Adsorption and irradiation of HCN alone (◊), adsorbed in olivine (O), adsorbed in serpentine (▲), and-irradiated at different doses.

A series of studies show that organic material was produced in high abundance from HCN at high radiation doses. The radiolytic products included gases (CO_2, NH_4, and CO) and oligomeric materials that release carboxylic acids (succinic, malonic, citric, and tricarballylic acids) and amino acids upon acid hydrolysis. These experiments suggest that minerals could have actively participated in chemical evolution processes

3. Final Remarks

Studies in radiation chemistry can provide a deeper insight into the chemical processes that may have importance for prebiotic chemistry. The chemical action of ionizing radiation is essential in producing reactive species. In a water dominant system, CN-containing compound radicals from the water decomposition react by addition/abstraction to the triple C-N bond and produced oligomers mainly as polyamides and polyesters. Upon hydrolysis, these oligomers released compounds of biological significance such as amino acids, carboxylic acids, purines, and some amines. The formation of these radiolytic products was observed at low RCN concentrations, low radiation doses, and in frozen solutions (77 K). The radiolytic behavior of HCN is affected by the presence of a solid surface by enhancing its chemical decomposition.

These results underline the importance of radiation-induced reactions in chemical evolution processes in the early Earth and in extraterrestrial environments, and of course, reinforce the role of HCN and in general, of the nitriles, in the chemical evolution processes that could accomplished on the early Earth or other bodies containing them, such as comets, the atmosphere of some planets, the interstellar matter and many other places in the Universe.

Acknowledgments

This study was supported by PAPIIT grant IN110712-3 and CONACyT grant 168579.

References

[1] Anderson, R. B. (1984). *The Fischer-Tropsch reaction* Academic Press, London.

[2] Bernal, J.D. (1951). *The physical bases of life*. Routlege and Keegan Paul. Londres. 80 pp.

[3] Birch, F. (1954). Heat from radioactivity. In *Nuclear Geology*, ed. H. Faul. New York: John Wiley.

[4] Boonman, A. M. S., Stark, R., van der Tak, F. F. S., van Dishoek, E. F., van der Wal, P. B., Shäfer, F., de Lange, G. and Laauwen, W. M

(2001). Highly abundant HCN in the inner hot envelope of GL 2591: probing the birth of a hot core? *Astrophys. Journal*. 553: L63-L67.

[5] Castric, P. (1981). The metabolism of hydrogen cyanide by bacteria. In: Vennesland, B., Conn, E. E., Knowles, C. J., Westley J. and F.Wissing (Eds). *Cyanide in Biology*. Academic Press. London.

[6] Chada, M. S., Lawless, J. G., Flores, J. J. and C. Ponnamperuma (1971). Experiments in Jovain atmospheres. In: Buvet, R. Ponnamperuma C. (Eds.). *Chemical Evolution and Origins of Life*. North Holland, Amsterdam.

[7] Colín-García, M., Negrón-Mendoza, A. and Ramos-Bernal, S., (2009). Organics produced by irradiation of frozen and liquid HCN solutions: implications for chemical evolution studies. *Astrobiology*. 9: 279-288.

[8] Could, P.E., (1977). Atmospheric and hydrospheric evolution on the primitive Earth. In: *The Archean Search for the Begining*. Mc all G.J.H. (Ed.). Dowden Hutchinson & Ross Inc. United States.

[9] Draganić, I., Draganić, Z., Petković, L., and Nikolić, A., (1973) Radiation chemistry of aqueous solutions of simple RCN [hydrogen or alkyl cyanide] compounds. *Journal of the American Chemical Society*. 95: 7193-7199.

[10] Draganić, Z. D., Draganić, I. G., and Jovanović, S. V., (1978). The radiation chemistry of aqueous solutions of cyanamide. *Radiation Research*. 75: 508-518.

[11] Draganić, I. G., Draganić, Z. D., and Vujošević, S., (1984a). Some radiation-chemical aspects of chemistry in cometary nuclei. *Icarus*. 60: 464-475.

[12] Draganić, Z. D; Draganić, I. G.; Azamar, J. A.; Negrón-Mendoza A. (1984b). Radiation-chemistry of over-irradiated aqueous-solutions of hydrogen-cyanide and ammonium cyanide. *Journal of Molecular Evolution*. 21: 356-363.

[13] Draganić, I. G. (2000) Radiation chemical approaches to chemical evolution processes, in *The role of radiation in the origin and evolution of the Earth,* Ed. Akaboshi, M., Fujii, N, and Navarro, R. Kyoto University Press, Kyoto, Japan.pp: 54-72.

[14] Duffey, S. S., (1981) Cyanide and arthropods. In: Vennesland, B., Conn, E. E., Knowles, C. J., Westley J. and F.Wissing (Eds). *Cyanide in Biology*. Academic Press. London.

[15] Ferris J. P. and Chen C. T. (1975). Chemical evolution. XXVI. Photochemistry of methane, nitrogen, and water mixtures as a model for

the atmosphere of the primitive earth. *Journal of the American Chemical Society*. 97: 2962–2967.

[16] Ferris, J. P. and Orgel, L. E. (1966). An unusual photochemical rearrangement in the synthesis of adenine from hydrogen cyanide. *Journal of the American Chemical Society*. 88:1074.

[17] Fry W. E. and Myers D. F., (1981) Hydrogen cyanide metabolism by fungal pathogens of cyanogenic plants. In: Vennesland, B., Conn, E. E., Knowles, C. J., Westley J. and F.Wissing (Eds). *Cyanide in Biology*. Academic Press. London.

[18] Fry W. E. and Evans P.H. (1977). Association of formamide hydro-lyase with fungal pathogenicity to cyanogenic plants. *Phytopathology*. 67: 1001-1006.

[19] Gerakines, P. A., Moore, M. H., and Hudson, R. L. (2004). Ultraviolet photolysis and proton irradiation of astrophysical ice analogs containing hydrogen cyanide. *Icarus*. 170: 202-213.

[20] Gupta, S., Ochiai, E., and Ponnamperuma, C., (1981). Organic synthesis in the atmosphere of Titan. *Nature*. 293: 725-727.

[21] Hawker Jr, Oró J. (1981). Cyanamide Mediated Synthesis of Peptides Containing Histidine and Hydrophobic Amino Acids. *Journal of Molecular. Evolution*. 17: 285-294.

[22] Ip, W. H., Balsiger, H., Geiss, J., Goldstein, B. E., Kettmann, G., Lazarus, A. J., Meier, A., Rosenbauer, H., and Schelley E. (1990). Giotto ISM measurements of the production rate of hydrogen cyanide in the coma of Comet Halley. *Annales Geophysicae*. 8: 319-325.

[23] Irvine, W.M., (1998) Extraterrestrial organic matter: a review. *Origins of Life and Evolution of the Biospheres*. 28: 365-383.

[24] Johansson, L. E. B., Andersson, C., Ellder, J., Friberg, P., Hjalmarson, A., Hoglund, B., Irvine, W. M., Olofsson, H., and Rydbeck, G., (1984). Spectral Scan of Orion-A and Irc + 10216 from 72 to 91 GHz. *Astronomy and Astrophysics*. 130: 227-256.

[25] Lazcano, A. and Miller S.L. (1994). How long did it take for life to begin and envolve to cyanobacteria? *Journal of Molecular Evolution*. 39: 546-554.

[26] Levy, M., Miller, S.L., and Oró, J., (1999) Production of Guanine from NH_4CN Polymerizations. *Journal of Molecular Evolution*. 49: 165-168.

[27] Levy, M., Miller, S. L., Brinton, K., and Bada, J. L. (2000). Prebiotic Synthesis of Adenine and Amino Acids under Europa-like Conditions, *Icarus*. 145: 609–613.

[28] Magee-Sauer K., Mumma M. J., DiSanti M. A., Russo N. D. and Rettig T.W. (1999). Infrared Spectroscopy of the ν3 Band of Hydrogen Cyanide in Comet C/1995 O1 Hale-Bopp. *Icarus*. 142: 498-598.
[29] Matthews, H. and Sears, T., (1986). Interstellar molecular line searches at 1.5 centimeters. *The Astrophysical Journal*. 300: 766-772.
[30] Matthews, C.N. and Minard, R.D., (2008). Hydrogen cyanide polymers connect cosmochemistry and biochemistry. *Organic Matter in Space, Proceedings IAU Symposium*. 251: 453-458.
[31] Matthews, C.N.M. and Moser, R. E., (1966). Prebiological protein synthesis. *Proceedings of the National Academy of Sciences*. 56: 1087-1094.
[32] Miller, S. L. (1953). A production of amino acids under possible primitive Earth Conditions. *Science*. 117: 528-529.
[33] Miller, S. and Orgel L. (1974). *The origins of life on the Earth*. Prentice Hall, Inc. New Jersey.
[34] Mosqueira, F. G., Albarrán, G. and Negrón-Mendoza, A. (1996). A review of conditions affecting the radiolysis due to ^{40}K on nucleic acid bases and their derivatives adsorbed on clay minerals: Implications in Prebiotic Chemistry. *Origins of Life and Evolution of the Biosphere*. 26: 75-94.
[35] Mukhin, L.M. (1974) Evolution of organic compounds in volcanic regions. *Nature*, 251: 50-51.
[36] Nartey, F. (1981). Cyanogenesis in tropical feeds and foodstuffs. In: Vennesland, B., Conn, E. E., Knowles, C. J., Westley J. and F.Wissing (Eds). *Cyanide in Biology*. Academic Press. London.
[37] Negrón-Mendoza, A., Ramos-Bernal, S. and Mosqueira, F. G. (2010). *Astrobiology: Emergence, search and detection of life*. Ed. V. Basiuk, American Scientific Publishers, Los Angeles, US.
[38] Negrón-Mendoza, A. and Albarrán G. (1993). Chemical effects of ionizing radiation and sonic energy in the context of chemical evolution. In Ponnamperuma, C. and Chela-Flores, J. (Eds). Chemical Evolution: *Origin of Life*. A. Deepak Publishing.
[39] Negrón-Mendoza A., Draganić, Z. D. (1984). Search for heterocyclic radiolytic products in aqueous solutions of cyanides, *Advances in Space Research*. 4: 121-124.
[40] Negrón-Mendoza, A and Ramos-Bernal, S., (1998). Radiolysis of carboxylic acids adsorbed in clay minerals. *Radiation Physics and Chemistry*. 52: 395-397.

[41] Oró J., Rewers, K., Odom D. ,(1982). Criteria for the emergence and evolution of life in the Solar system. *Origins of Life*. 12: 285-305.

[42] Oró, J. and Kimball, A. P., (1961). Synthesis of purines under possible primitive Earth conditions. I. Adenine from hydrogen cyanide. *Archives of Biochemistry and Biophysics* 94: 217-227.

[43] Ponnamperuma, C. and Mack, R., (1965). Nucleotide synthesis under possible primitive Earth conditions. *Science*. 148: 1221-1223.

[44] Schopf, J. M. and Packer B. M., (1987). Early Achaean (3.3 billion year-old) Microfossils from Warrawoona Group, Australia. *Science*. 237: 70-73.

[45] Spinks, J. W. T. and R. J. Woods. (1990). *An introduction to Radiation Chemistry*. Wiley-Interscience Publication. New York.

[46] Stern, A.S., (2003). The evolution of comets in the Oort cloud and Kuiper belt. *Nature*. 424: 639-642.

[47] Steudel, A., Batenburg, L. F., Fischer, H. R., Weidler, P. G., and Emmerich, K., (2009) Alteration of swelling clay minerals by acid activation. *Applied Clay Science*. 44: 105-115.

[48] Trimble, V. (1997). Origin of the Biologically Important Elements. *Origins of Life and Evolution of the Biosphere*. 27: 3-21.

[49] Toupance, G., Bossard, A., and Raulin F. (1978). Far UV irradiation of model prebiotic atmospheres. In: H. Noda (Ed.). *Origin of Life*. JSSP, Tokio. Pp. 159-165.

[50] Vuitton, V., Yelle, R. V., and Anicich, V. G., (2006) The Nitrogen Chemistry of Titan's Upper Atmosphere Revealed. *The Astrophysical Journal Letters*. 647, L175.

[51] Woeller, F. and Ponnamperuma, C., (1969) Organic synthesis in a simulated Jovian atmosphere. *Icarus*. 10: 386-392.

In: Cyanide
Editor: Benito Soto-Blanco
ISBN: 978-1-62618-297-4

Chapter 2

CYANIDE POISONING IN ANIMALS AND HUMANS

Antônio Carlos Lopes Câmara[a] and Benito Soto-Blanco[b]
[a]Veterinary Hospital, Universidade Federal Rural do Semi-árido (UFERSA), Mossoró, RN, Brazil
[b]Department of Veterinary Clinics and Surgery, Universidade Federal de Minas Gerais (UFMG), Belo Horizonte, MG, Brazil

ABSTRACT

Cyanide is a ubiquitous substance in the environment. It can be released from cyanogenic plants, industrial processes (such as metal processing, electroplating, and acrylic and chemical synthesis), and medicinal drugs (such as nitroprusside). Cyanide inhibits several cellular enzymes, including cytochrome oxidase, which is a key enzyme in the cellular respiratory chain. Most of the cyanide absorbed by an organism is detoxified by enzymatic combination with sulfur, and acute poisoning occurs when detoxification systems are overwhelmed. Acute cyanide poisoning is potentially fatal and is a result of cellular hypoxia and cytotoxic anoxia. Long-term exposure to cyanide is responsible for various toxic effects, including reduced weight gain, damage to the liver, impaired thyroid function, and neuropathies. Furthermore, various experimental studies and field cases in several animal species have verified that exposure to cyanide or to cyanogenic plants results in reproductive disturbances.

INTRODUCTION

Cyanide is one of the most studied substances in toxicology due to its very high toxicity (Osweiler et al. 1985; Salkowski and Penney, 1994). Cyanide poisoning has been known to occur since ancient times. In ancient Egypt, cyanogenic plant extracts were used for the execution of death sentences. The Roman conquerors learned how to manipulate cyanide when they invaded Egypt, and this substance was used in many murders throughout the Roman Empire. In 1782, Charles Guillaume Scheele, one of the founders of organic chemistry, determined the presence of cyanide in plants; while in 1814, Louis Gay-Lussac was the first person to isolate a cyanogenic glycoside. However, the mechanism of action underlying the toxicity of cyanide was not determined until 1927, when it was discovered by Warburg Iorsque (Paulet, 1960).

Cyanide is released by several processes, including acrylic and ammonia manufacturing, electroplating, steel production, the extraction of gold and silver, and jewelry polishing (El Ghawabi et al., 1975; Blanc et al., 1985; Salkowski and Penney, 1994; Coentrão and Moura, 2011). Hydrocyanic acid is also found in smoke, and it is generated by the incomplete combustion of carbon compounds in fires, cigarettes and propulsion motors (ATSDR, 1993; Alarie, 2002; Stefanidou and Athanaselis, 2004; Grabowska et al., 2012; Youso et al., 2012). Because the number of smokers worldwide is in the hundreds of millions, cigarette smoking represents an important source of exposure to cyanide (ATSDR, 1993; Youso et al., 2012). Cyanide is commonly used to commit suicide (Winek et al., 1978; Gill et al., 2004; Bebarta et al., 2011; Garlich et al., 2012) and homicide (Vycudilik and Gmeiner, 2009), and it may be used as a chemical warfare agent (Szinicz, 2005; Rodgers and Condurache, 2010). Cyanide poisoning can also occur through the diet and is caused almost exclusively by glycosides present in plants, such as cassava, apple, and peach (Poulton, 1983; Barceloux, 2009; Blagbrough et al., 2010). Additionally, there are potentially toxic drugs that release cyanide, including laetrile (amygdalin), which has been used as a treatment for cancer (Huxtable, 1990; Milazzo et al., 2007, 2011), and sodium nitroprusside, a potent hypotensive agent (Schulz et al., 1982; Schulz, 1984).

The main sources of cyanide-induced animal poisoning are cyanogenic plants (Poulton, 1983; Soto-Blanco et al., 2001a). Collective intoxication of animals by cyanide from mining and industrial effluents has also been described (Berlier et al., 1973; Henny et al. 1994; Aslani et al., 2004). Intentional cases of cyanide poisoning may also occur in animals.

CYANIDE IN PLANTS

The accumulation of cyanide is very common in plants. In fact, the number of cyanogenic plants was estimated to be at least 2,500 species (Vetter, 2000). The most probable function of the production of cyanogenic glycosides by plant tissues is as a plant defense mechanism in order to minimize herbivore predation (Jones, 1998).

Two groups of products of plant metabolism, the cyanogenic glycosides and cyanolipids, release hydrocyanic acid through the action of hydroxylases. Of these two groups, the cyanogenic glycosides are the most important, with more than 25 types identified (Poulton, 1983; Cheeke, 1998). Examples of cyanogenic glycosides include: amygdalin, isolated from the Rosaceae family (e.g., apple, pear and cherry); dhurrin, present in plants of the genus *Sorghum* (e.g., grain sorghum and Sudan grass); and linamarin, which is produced by cassava, white clover and flax (Cheeke and Shull, 1985; Cheeke, 1998).

The release of cyanide from glycosides occurs in two steps through the action of endogenous plant enzymes, as shown in Figure 1. In the first reaction, the β-glycosidase enzyme catalyzes the breakdown of carbohydrates and the cyanohydrin or aglycone moieties. Cyanohydrin is then dissociated by the hydroxynitrile lyase enzyme, hydrocyanic acid and aldehydes or ketones (Conn, 1978; Cheeke and Shull, 1985; Osweiler et al., 1985; Cheeke, 1998).

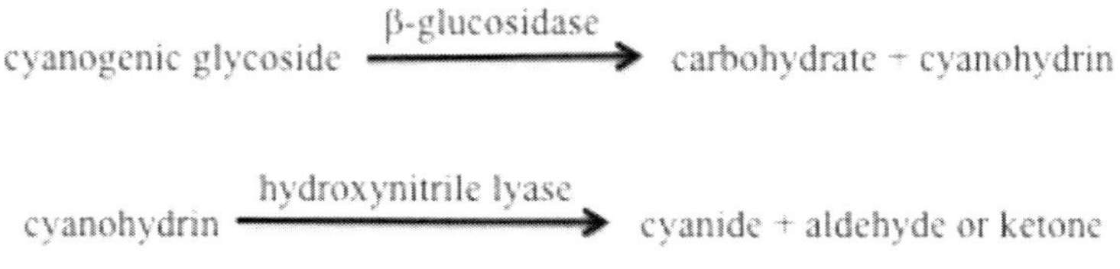

Figure 1. Breakdown reactions of cyanogenic glycosides for cyanidric acid (HCN) release.

In the intact plant cell, cyanide is not liberated due to a spatial separation of the cyanogenic glycosides, which are located in the vacuoles, and the degrading enzymes, which are located in the cytosol. Physical damage to plant cells promotes the combination of the glycosides and the enzymes and the consequent release of cyanide (Conn, 1978; Cheeke and Shull, 1985; Osweiler et al. 1985; Cheeke, 1998). Therefore, conditions that result in plant damage, such as drying, freezing or wilting, increase the toxicity of the plant at the time of ingestion (Osweiler et al. 1985). Furthermore, the enzymes that hydrolyze the cyanogenic glycosides are also produced by ruminal bacteria (Majak and Cheng, 1984; Majak et al., 1990). Great variation was found in the activities of the ruminal hydrolytic enzymes, with some animals possessing more efficient mechanisms for releasing cyanide from plants than others (Majak et al., 1980; Majak, 1992; Soto-Blanco et al., 2008). In monogastric organisms, these glycosides are also hydrolyzed by both intestinal bacteria (Fomunyam et al., 1984; Frakes et al., 1986) and hydrochloric acid present in the stomach (Conn, 1978).

The factors that influence the toxicity of cyanogenic plants are: the concentration of the compound in the plant, the amount of plant ingested, animal species, speed of ingestion, types of food eaten simultaneously, the presence of active degrading enzymes in plants and the gastrointestinal tract, and the ability of the animal to detoxify cyanide (Conn, 1978; Osweiler et al., 1985; Lopez et al., 1992). Another possible factor influencing the toxicity of cyanogenic plants may be metabolic tolerance. Animals continuously exposed to cyanogenic plants may develop some resistance (Shaw, 1986). However, the development of this tolerance was brought into question (Soto-Blanco et al., 2005).

TOXICOKINETICS AND MECHANISM OF ACTION

Cyanide is readily absorbed by the mucous membranes and is quickly detoxified (Schulz, 1984; Sousa et al., 2003). Most of the absorbed cyanide (approximately 80%) is converted into thiocyanate. This reaction is catalyzed by the rhodanese enzyme (thiosulfate sulfurtransferase, EC 2.8.1.1), which requires thiosulfate as a source of sulfur (Sorbo, 1951, 1953; Bahri, 1988; Sousa et al., 2003), as shown in Figure 2. A small portion of the adsorbed cyanide undergoes conjugation with cysteine to form 2-imino-4-thiazolidine-carboxylic acid and 2-iminothiazoline-4-carboxylic acid, and with hydroxycobalamin (vitamin B_{12}) to form cyanocobalamin. Formic acid may also be formed in small amounts. A fraction of the absorbed cyanide is eliminated by the lungs in the form of HCN (Ansell and Lewis, 1970).

$$S_2O_3^{2-} + CN^- \xrightarrow{\text{rhodanese}} SO_3^{2-} + SCN^-$$

Figure 2. Conversion of a cyanide ion (CN^-) into thiocyanate (SCN^-) by the rhodanese enzyme using thiosulfate ($S_2O_3^{2-}$) as a sulfur donor.

Cyanide inhibits the action of enzymes that contain metals, especially iron. The most important enzyme inhibited by cyanide is cytochrome oxidase, which is a key enzyme in the cellular respiratory chain (Ballantyne, 1987). Trivalent iron (Fe^{3+}) from the cytochrome oxidase enzyme reacts with cyanide complexes to form cytochrome oxidase-CN. This reaction maintains the iron in the trivalent form and drops the electron transport system and the respiratory chain, resulting in cytotoxic hypoxia and anoxia. The highest levels of cytochrome oxidase are found in tissues with high oxidative metabolism, such as the central nervous system (CNS) and cardiac musculature (Way, 1984; Osweiler et al., 1985).

Cyanide is also involved in the production of free radicals in neurons, resulting in lipid peroxidation and cell damage (Johnson et al., 1987; Ardelt et al., 1989, 1994; Müller and Krieglstein, 1995; Gunasekar et al., 1996, 1998; Mills et al., 1996; Kanthasamy et al., 1997; Yamamoto and Tang, 1998). Furthermore, cyanide inhibits both the catalase (Kamalu, 1995; Gunasekar et al., 1996, 1998; Kanthasamy et al., 1997) and glutathione peroxidase enzymes (Elzubeir and Davis, 1990; Gutzwiller, 1993; Davis et al., 1996). Other authors (Gunasekar et al., 1996, 1998, Sun et al. 1997; Yamamoto and Tang, 1998) have suggested that cyanide promotes the activation of N-methyl-D-aspartate (NMDA), generating an influx of calcium ions, glutamate release and the formation of free radicals. Cyanide also interferes with several neurotransmitters, including γ-aminobutyric acid (GABA) (Tursky and Sajter, 1962; Cassel et al., 1991), glutamic acid (Cassel et al., 1991), acetylcholine (Owasoya and Iramain, 1980), dopamine (Cassel et al., 1995), excitatory amino acids (McCaslin and Yu, 1992; Gunasekar et al., 1996) and nitric oxide (Gunasekar et al., 1996).

ACUTE CYANIDE TOXICITY

Acute toxicity occurs when the amounts of cyanide absorbed greatly exceed the minimum concentration required to inhibit cytochrome oxidase. Furthermore, acute toxicity is promoted when the amount of cyanide is greater than that supported by detoxification enzymes (Way, 1984).

The lethal intravenous dose of HCN in sheep and goats was established to be approximately 2 mg/kg body weight when administered rapidly, and 3.9 mg/kg when administered slowly. For cattle, a lethal intravenous dose is approximately 2 mg/kg in young animals, and 4 to 5 mg/kg in adult animals (Saad and Camargo, 1967). The lethal dose of potassium cyanide (KCN) in dogs was estimated to be 2.4 mg/kg (Ivankovich et al., 1980). In humans, it is believed that the lethal oral dose is approximately 100 mg of HCN, 150 mg of sodium cyanide (NaCN), and 200 mg of KCN (Salkowski and Penney, 1994).

The clinical signs of acute cyanide poisoning include paresis, generalized muscle spasms and excitement. Initially, the respiratory rate is increased, followed by dyspnea that progresses to respiratory arrest. Mucous membranes are bright, and the eyes display mydriasis (Osweiler et al., 1985; Oruc et al., 2006; Nicholson, 2012). Lactic acidosis with hyperglycemia occurs to varying degrees as a consequence of increased anaerobic metabolism (Katsumata et al., 1980; Salkowski and Penney, 1995; Baud et al., 2002; Oruc et al., 2006). The animal may develop convulsions, which may be followed by death. When the cyanide concentration absorbed is lethal, death generally occurs within minutes of the onset of clinical signs (Osweiler et al., 1985; Nicholson, 2012).

At necropsy, the findings are not pathognomonic. Venous blood may be bright red because oxygen is not released from red blood cells for cellular respiration. Clotting is often slow or incomplete (Maxie and Youssef, 2007; Nicholson, 2012). The lungs and trachea may become congested, and there might be subendocardial hemorrhage and subepicardial petechiae, which suggest agonal death. The abomasum and intestines may also be congested, with the presence of petechiae, and the characteristic odor of cyanide (bitter almond odor) may be noted in the ruminal content (Osweiler et al., 1985; Nicholson, 2012). Histological examination of the brain may show degenerative lesions, mainly in the gray or white matter (Maxie and Youssef, 2007).

Prolonged Cyanide Toxicity

Prolonged exposure to cyanide has been associated with a number of pathologies, including impaired growth, hypothyroidism, pancreatic diabetes, nervous disorders, and reproductive disturbances. Furthermore, KCN promoted mild degenerative damage to hepatocytes in rabbits (Okolie and Osagie, 1999), rats (Sousa et al., 2002), goats (Soto-Blanco et al., 2005, 2008), pigs (Manzano et al., 2007), and quail (Rocha-e-Silva et al., 2010), and the degeneration of renal tubular epithelial cells in rabbits (Okolie and Osagie, 1999), rats (Sousa et al., 2002), and pigs (Manzano et al., 2007).

Impaired Growth

Body weight is one of the main evaluation parameters in toxicology, often indicating the early onset of the toxic effects of a substance in animals (Stevens and Gallo, 1989). Several studies have associated chronic cyanide intoxication with reduced body weight gain in broilers (Panigrahi et al., 1992), rats (Guzmán et al., 1977; Philbrick et al., 1979; Akanji and Fumuyiwa, 1993), dogs (Ibebunjo et al., 1992), pigs (Tewe et al., 1984), sheep (Onwuka et al., 1992), and goats (Onwuka, 1992; Onwuka et al., 1992), as well as in humans who have been occupationally exposed to cyanide (Blanc et al., 1985).

In addition to decreased weight gain, animals receiving 3.0 mg/kg KCN had lower overall weights and carcass yields. The observed effects on weight gain and carcass indicate that cyanide promoted changes in lipid metabolism and protein content in these animals. In fact, Ibebunjo et al. (1992) observed a greater deposition of fat in the subcutaneous tissue, as well as reduced muscle development, in dogs that were chronically exposed to cyanide. The observed reduction in muscle development may have resulted from the depletion of amino acids containing sulfur, which serves to detoxify cyanide because endogenous sulfate is not sufficient to withstand this reaction (Onwuka et al., 1992). Another hypothesis is that this result is a consequence of the reduction in plasma levels of T3 in hypothyroidism because both the secretion of growth hormone (Lloyd et al., 1990) and the number of receptors for this hormone are reduced (Koenig et al., 1987).

Hypothyroidism

One pathological consequence that has been associated with chronic exposure to cyanide is hypothyroidism. Hypothyroidism was observed in rats (Tewe et al., 1977; Barrett et al., 1978; Philbrick et al., 1979), rabbits (Ratnakumar and Rajan, 1992), dogs (Kamalu and Agharanya, 1991), pigs (Tewe et al., 1984; Oke, 1984; Ong, 1989), sheep (Gutzwiller, 1993) and also in humans (Adewusi and Akindahunsi, 1994; Gaitan et al., 1994). The main product of the transformation of cyanide, thiocyanate, is a known goitrogenic compound. Thiocyanate competes with the iodine protein carrier in the thyroid gland, decreasing iodine uptake and thereby inhibiting the production of thyroid hormones (Maloof and Soodak, 1959; Wollman, 1962; Greer et al., 1966; Scranton et al., 1969; Carrasco, 1993; Delange and Ermans, 1996). It is known that these hormones act on metabolism, growth and cell differentiation, especially in the CNS and cellular metabolic processes (Kaneko, 2008). Thus, all of these functions are compromised in the case of hypothyroidism.

It was also verified that selenium (Se) deficiency results from chronic cyanide intake in several animal species, including birds (Elzubeir and Daves, 1990; Davis et al., 1996), rats (Beilstein and Whanger, 1984) and sheep (Gutzwiller, 1993). Se is essential for the synthesis of the type I 5'-deiodinase enzyme, which performs the peripheral conversion of thyroxine (T_4) to the active hormone triiodothyronine (T_3). In selenium deficiency, synthesis is impaired, and there is a consequent reduction in the activity of this enzyme (Berry and Larsen, 1994; St. Germain and Galton, 1997). The exact mechanism of cyanide-induced selenium deficiency is not fully understood. It is known that selenium excretion in rats is increased in chronic cyanide poisoning (Beilstein and Whanger, 1984). In the rumen, selenium joins with cyanide to form a compound that is poorly absorbed (Gutzwiller, 1993).

Histopathological examination of the thyroid glands from cyanide-treated animals revealed increased amounts of resorption vacuoles in the colloid of thyroid follicles (Soto-Blanco et el., 2001a, 2005, 2008; Manzano et al., 2007; Rocha-e-Silva et al., 2010). Resorption vacuoles are associated with increased secretory activity of the thyroid gland, which is a probable response to impaired thyroid function. They were also present in the work of Bahri (1987), in goats experimentally fed cassava leaves, and Marques et al. (1985), in goats fed with plants of the *Brassica* genus (rich thiocyanate). Although this finding is not described in either study, it can easily be observed in the pictures of the thyroid presented.

Pancreatic Diabetes

Several studies have linked the intake of cassava and other foods containing cyanogenic glycosides to the development of pancreatic diabetes, also referred to by some authors as tropical diabetes. Thus, it is believed that through pancreatic acinar lesions, injury occurs in the islets of Langerhans, thereby causing diabetes (McMillan and Geevarghese, 1979; Davidson, 1980; Assan et al., 1988; Pitchumoni et al., 1988; Kamalu, 1991, 1995; Petersen, 2002). In fact, studies conducted in humans who regularly eat improperly detoxified cassava revealed high incidences of pancreatic diabetes, and individuals affected with this disease were treated with high doses of insulin. Histopathologic findings revealed the presence of calcium crystals in the pancreatic parenchyma (McMillan and Geevarghese, 1979; Davidson, 1980).

In a study conducted on dogs fed a cassava-based diet for 14 weeks, we observed an increase in gluconeogenesis from protein, as well as increased blood insulin levels. Histopathology revealed hemorrhage, necrosis, fibrosis and atrophy of acinar tissue, as well as fibrosis of the islets of Langerhans (Kamalu, 1991).

The role of cyanide and cyanogenic plants in the etiology of pancreatic diabetes has been contested (Soto-Blanco et al., 2001b). Administration of cyanide to several animal species resulted in no changes in plasma glucose levels and no histological lesions in the pancreas (Soto-Blanco et al., 2001b, 2002a, 2008, 2009; Manzano et al., 2007; Rocha-e-Silva et al., 2010). Some authors (Kamalu, 1991, 1995; Akanji and Famuyiwa, 1993) suggest that this organ injury may be related to the effects of linamarin, a cyanogenic glycoside present in cassava, and not to cyanide. This mechanism may be produced by inhibiting the $Na^{+}K^{+}$ ATPase enzyme with intact linamarin (Kamalu, 1995). However, the administration of cyanogenic plants did not produce any diabetogenic effects (Soto-Blanco et al., 2008). Furthermore, several other authors performed epidemiological studies and found no correlation between the development of diabetes in humans and the consumption of cassava (Mohan et al., 1985; Cooles, 1988; Richens and Wesseling, 1988; Vannasaeng et al., 1988; Chari et al., 1992; Kiatsayompoo et al., 1993; Narendranathan and Cheriyan, 1994).

Nervous Disorders

In humans, chronic exposure to cyanide has been associated with the etiology of various nervous diseases, such as tropical ataxic neuropathy (Osuntokun et al., 1969; Osuntokun, 1981; Njoh, 1990), konzo (Tylleskär et al., 1991, 1995; Banea et al., 1997; Nzwalo and Cliff, 2001), tobacco amblyopia (Heaton et al., 1958), retrolobular neuritis (Moore, 1934; Freeman and Heaton, 1961) and Leber's optic atrophy (Wilson, 1965; Adams et al., 1966; Freeman, 1988).

Both tropical ataxic neuropathy and konzo are pathologies that are related to prolonged exposure to cyanide from a diet where inadequately detoxified cassava is a staple and protein consumption is low. Tropical ataxic neuropathy is characterized by myelopathy, bilateral optic atrophy, polyneuropathy and bilateral hearing loss. In addition, Parkinson's disease, cerebellar disintegration, psychosis and dementia have also been associated with this disease (Monekosso and Annan, 1964; Osuntokun, 1968, 1981, Makene and

Wilson, 1972). In contrast, konzo is an upper motor neuron disorder characterized by the sudden onset of permanent and non-progressive spastic paraparesis, without any neurological manifestation (Tylleskär et al., 1991, 1995; Banea et al., 1997).

Field observations in horses, cattle and sheep grazing on *Sorghum* spp, a cyanogenic plant, revealed a neurologic dysfunction characterized by posterior ataxia, or staggering, and permanent urinary incontinence (Adams et al., 1969; McKenzie and McMicking, 1977; Morgan et al., 1990; Bradley et al., 1995; Odrizola, 2011). The predominant pathological findings in horses and cattle were Wallerian degeneration and demyelination in the white matter of the spinal cord (Adams et al., 1969; McKenzie and McMicking, 1977). In sheep, the main findings were the presence of spheroids in the proximal segments of axons at the nuclei of the medulla, cerebellum, and midbrain (Bradley et al., 1995). However, it is uncertain whether cyanide is responsible for this dysfunction.

Experimental reports in several animal species chronically treated with cyanide have described central nervous system (CNS) lesions. Studies conducted on rats have found that high doses of cyanide administered chronically to these animals produced CNS lesions, including the degeneration of neurons in the hippocampus and cortex and the Purkinje cells in the cerebellum (Smith et al., 1963; Soto-Blanco et al., 2002a), the presence of spheroids on the ventral horn of the spinal cord, the loss of cerebellar white matter (Soto-Blanco et al., 2002a), and vacuolation and gliosis in the spinal cord and white matter (Philbrick et al., 1979). An experimental study carried out on mice subjected to prolonged treatment with KCN found lesions mainly in the substantia nigra and cortex (Mills et al., 1999).

In goats treated with KCN and the cyanogenic plant *Prunus virginiana* (chokecherry), nervous system tissue had spongiosis and spheroids in the mesencephalon (Soto-Blanco et al., 2008). In another study, goats treated chronically with KCN developed axonal dystrophy (spheroids) and spongiosis and gliosis in the medulla oblongata, gliosis in the pons and Purkinje cell degeneration in the cerebellum (Soto-Blanco et al., 2002b). Degeneration of cerebellar white matter and Purkinje cells were observed in pigs dosed with KCN (Manzano et al., 2007). Furthermore, spongiosis was evident in the mesencephalon of quail dosed with cyanide (Rocha-e-Silva et al., 2010).

Although several studies have been conducted on the toxicity of cyanide in the CNS, little is known about the underlying mechanism. Some studies indicate that the neurotoxic effects of cyanide may be related to the cellular production of free radicals, resulting in lipid peroxidation and neuronal damage (Johnson et al., 1987; Ardelt et al., 1989, 1994; Müller and Krieglstein, 1995; Gunasekar et al., 1996, 1998; Mills et al., 1996; Kanthasamy et al., 1997; Yamamoto and Tang, 1998). Furthermore, cyanide inhibits catalase (Kamalu, 1995; Gunasekar et al., 1996, 1998; Kanthasamy et al., 1997) and glutathione peroxidase (Elzubeir and Davis, 1990; Gutzwiller, 1993; Davis et al., 1996). Therefore, although it has been recognized that free radicals are related to this toxic effect, the mechanism underlying the formation of these radicals remains unknown. Kamalu (1995) suggested that chronic cyanide intoxication would generate cycles of hypoxia/normoxia by inhibiting the cytochrome oxidase enzyme, immediately reversing the transformation of this toxic agent to thiocyanate. These cycles would result in the generation of free radicals. Moreover, other authors (Gunasekar et al., 1996, 1998, Sun et al. 1997; Yamamoto and Tang, 1998) have suggested that cyanide promotes the activation of N-methyl-D-aspartate (NMDA), generating an influx of calcium ions that is responsible for glutamate release and the formation of free radicals. McCaslin and Yu (1992) have suggested that the formation of free radicals would result in the kainate-induced release of glutamate and taurine but would not result in NMDA-induced release. Furthermore, some studies related free radical formation to the release of nitric oxide in the CNS (Baskin et al., 1996a,b; Gunasekar et al., 1998; Yamamoto and Tang, 1998).

Another effect related to the neurotoxicity of this substance is the promotion of changes to the phospholipid membranes via activation of the phospholipase A2 enzyme (Yang et al., 1994). Furthermore, cyanide interferes with several neurotransmitters, including γ-aminobutyric acid (GABA) (Tursky and Sajter, 1962; Cassel et al., 1991), glutamic acid (Cassel et al., 1991), acetylcholine (Owasoya and Iramain, 1980), dopamine (Cassel et al., 1995), excitatory amino acids (McCaslin and Yu, 1992; Gunasekar et al., 1996) and nitric oxide (Gunasekar et al., 1996). Despite numerous studies directly indicating that cyanide is the main compound responsible for the toxic effects observed at the CNS level, Bitner et al. (1995, 1997) observed that 2-iminothiazolidine-4-carboxylic acid, a transformation product of the conjugation of cyanide with cysteine, has excitotoxic properties and causes selective loss of pyramidal neurons in the CA-1 region of the hippocampus.

Reproductive Disturbances

Various experimental studies and field cases have reported that exposure to cyanide or to cyanogenic plants was associated with reproductive disturbances, including lower body weight at birth, malformations and abortion. Mares and ewes fed cyanogenic crops or from cyanogenic pastures exhibited an increased incidence of miscarriage and skeletal defects in the offspring (Adams et al., 1969; Bradley et al., 1995). The occurrence of fetal malformations was experimentally reproduced in laboratory rodents treated with laetrile (Willhite, 1982) and the cyanogenic glycoside linamarin (Frakes et al., 1985). In contrast, no malformations were found in rats (Tewe et al., 1977; Sousa et al., 2007) and goats (Soto-Blanco and Górniak, 2004; Soto-Blanco et al., 2009) receiving cyanide during pregnancy.

The administration of cyanide to pregnant goats resulted in the placenta of one goat presenting an increased cotyledon surface area occupied by vascular lumina. Histological lesions in KCN-treated dams consisted of vacuolation of hepatocytes and thyroid follicular cells, an increased number of vacuoles on the thyroid follicular colloid, and spongiosis of the cerebral, internal capsule, and cerebellar peduncle tracts. Fetuses from these mothers showed vacuolation of hepatocytes and thyroid follicular cells and the formation of spheroids in the cerebellar white matter (Soto-Blanco et al., 2009).

References

Adams, JH; Blackwood, W; Wilson, J. Further clinical and pathological observations on Leber's optic atrophy. *Brain* 1966;89:15-26.

Adams, LG; Dollahite, JW; Romane, WM; Bullard, TL; Bridges, CH. Cystitis and ataxia associated with Sorghum ingestion by horses. *J Am Vet Med Assoc* 1969;155:518-524.

Adewusi, SRA; Akindahunsi, AA. Cassava processing, consumption, and cyanide toxicity. *J Toxicol Environ Health* 1994;43:13-23.

Akanji, AO; Famuyiwa, OO. The effects of chronic cassava consumption, cyanide intoxication and protein malnutrition on glucose tolerance in growing rats. *Br J Nutr* 1993;69:269-276.

Alarie, Y. Toxicity of fire smoke. *Crit Rev Toxicol* 2002;32:259-289.

Ansell, M; Lewis, FAS. A review of cyanide concentrations found in human organs. *J Forensic Med* 1970;17:148-155.

Ardelt, BK; Borowitz, JL; Isom, GE. Brain lipid peroxidation and antioxidant protectant mechanisms following acute cyanide intoxication. *Toxicology* 1989;56:147-154.

Ardelt, BK; Borowitz, JL; Maduh, EU; Swain, SL; Isom, GE. Cyanide-induced lipid peroxidation in different organs: subcellular distribution and hydroperoxide generation in neuronal cells. *Toxicology* 1994;89:127-137.

ATSDR – Agency for Toxic Substances and Disease Registry. Cyanide toxicity. *American Family Physician* 1993;48:107-114.

Aslani, MR; Mohri, M; Maleki, M; Sharifi, K; Mohammadi, GR; Chamsaz, M. Mass cyanide intoxication in sheep. *Vet Human Toxicol* 2004;46:186-187.

Assan, R; Assan, D; Thiebaut, MF; Laloux, S; Clauser, E; Boukersi, A. Diabetogenic tropical pancreatitis. *Diabetes Metab* 1988;14:299-312.

Bahri, S. Chronic effect of cassava leaves on the plasma thiocyanate and on the performance of the goat thyroid gland. *Penyakit Hewan* 1987;19(34)88-90.

Bahri; S. A study of detoxification of cyanide into thiocyanate in goats. *Penyakit Hewan* 1988;20(35)34-37.

Ballantyne, B. Toxicology of cyanides. In: Ballantyne, B; Marrs, TC, editors. Clinical and Experimental Toxicology of Cyanides. Bristol: Wright, 1987. p.41-126.

Banea, M; Tylleskär, T; Rosling, H. Konzo and Ebola in Bandundu region of Zaire. *Lancet* 1997;349(9052):621.

Barceloux, DG. Cyanogenic foods (cassava, fruit kernels, and cycad seeds). *Dis Mon* 2009;55:336-352.

Barrett, MDP; Alexander, JC; Hill, DC. Effect of linamarin on thiocyanate production and thyroid activity in rats. *J Toxicol Environ Health* 1978;4:735-740.

Baskin, SI; Nealley, EW; Lempka, JC. Cyanide toxicity in mice pretreated with diethylamine nitric oxide complex. *Human Exp Toxicol* 1996a;15:13-18.

Baskin, SI; Nealley, EW; Lempka, JC. The effects of EDRF/NO releasers or calcium ionophore A23187 on cyanide toxicity in mice. *Toxicol Appl Pharmacol* 1996b;139:349-355.

Baud, FJ; Borron, SW; Mégarbane, B; Trout, H; Lapostolle, F; Vicaut, E; Debray, M; Bismuth, C. Value of lactic acidosis in the assessment of the severity of acute cyanide poisoning. *Crit Care Med* 2002;30:2044-2050.

Beilstein, MA; Whanger, PD. Effects of cyanide on selenium metabolism in rats. *J Nutr* 1984;114:929-937.

Bebarta, VS; Pitotti, RL; Borys, DJ; Morgan, DL. Seven years of cyanide ingestions in the USA: Critically ill patients are common, but antidote use is not. *Emerg Med J* 2011;28:155-158.

Berlier, MM; Delatour; Falcoz; Lorgue; Mogeon. Trois cas d'intoxications collectives d'animaux domestiques dus à une pollution industrielle par les cyanures. *Bulletin de la Société des Sciences Vétérinaires et de Médecine Comparée de Lyon* 1973;71:49-50.

Berry, MJ; Larsen, PR. Selenocysteine and the structure, function, and regulation of iodothyronine deiodination: update 1994. *Endocrine Rev* 1994;3:265-269.

Bitner, RS; Kanthasamy, A; Isom, GE; Yim, GKW. Seizures and selective CA-1 hippocampal lesions induced by an excitotoxic cyanide metabolite, 2-iminothiazolidine-4-carboxylic acid. *NeuroToxicology* 1995;16:115-122.

Bitner, RS; Yim, GKW; Isom, GE. 2-iminothiazolidine-4-carboxylic acid produces hippocampal CA1 lesions independent of seizure excitation and glutamate receptor activation. *NeuroToxicology* 1997;18:191-200.

Blagbrough, IS; Bayoumi, SAL; Rowan, MG; Beeching, JR. Cassava: An appraisal of its phytochemistry and its biotechnological prospects. *Phytochemistry* 2010;71:1940-1951.

Blanc, P; Hogan, M; Mallin, K; Hryhorczuk, D; Hessl, S; Bernard, B. Cyanide intoxication among silver-reclaiming workers. *J Am Med Assoc* 1985;253:367-371.

Bradley, GA; Metcalf, HC; Reggiardo, C; Noon, TH; Bicknell, EJ; Lozano-Alarcon, F; Reed, RE; Riggs, MW. Neuroaxonal degeneration in sheep grazing *Sorghum* pastures. *J Vet Diag Invest* 1995;7:229-236.

Carrasco, N. Iodide transport in the thyroid gland. *Biochim Biophys Acta* 1993;1154:65-82.

Cassel, G; Karlsson, L; Sellstrom, A. On the inhibition of glutamic acid decarboxylase and gamma-aminobutyric acid transaminase by sodium cyanide. *Pharmacol Toxicol* 1991;69:238-241.

Cassel, GE; Koch, M; Tiger, G. The effects of cyanide on the extracellular levels of dopamine, 3,4-dihydroxyphenylacetic acid, homovanillic acid, 5-hydroxyindoleacetic acid and inositol phospholipid breakdown in the brain. *NeuroToxicology* 1995;16:73-82.

Chari, ST; Mohan, V; Jayanthi, V; Snehalatha, C; Malathi, S; Viswanathan, M; Madanagopalan, N. Comparative study of the clinical profiles of alcoholic chronic pancreatitis and tropical chronic pancreatitis in Tamil Nadu, south India. *Pancreas* 1992;7:52-58.

Cheeke, PR. Toxins intrinsic to cereal grains and other concentrate feeds. In: *Natural Toxicants in Feeds, Forages, and Poisonous Plants, 2nd edn.* Danville: Interstate Publishers, 1998. p.137-162.

Cheeke, PR; Shull, LR. Glycosides. In*: Natural Toxicants in Feeds and Poisonous Plants*. Westport: Avi, 1985. p.173-234.

Coentrão, L; Moura, D. Acute cyanide poisoning among jewelry and textile industry workers. *Am J Emerg Med* 2011;29:79-81.

Conn, EE. Cyanogenesis, the production of hidrogen cyanide, by plants. In: Keeler, RF; Van Kampen, KR; James, LF, editors. *Effects of Poisonous Plants on Livestock.* New York: Academic Press, 1978. p.301-310.

Cooles, P. Diabetes and cassava in Dominica. *Trop Geograph Med* 1988;40:272-273.

Davidson, JC. Dietary cyanide and tropical malnutrition diabetes. *Diabetes Care* 1980;3:703.

Davis, RH; Fear, J; Winton, AC. Interactions between dietary selenium, copper and sodium nitroprusside, a source of cyanide in growing chicks and laying hens. *Br Poult Sci* 1996;37:87-94.

Delange, FM; Ermans, AM. Iodine deficiency. In: Braverman, LE; Utiger, RD, editors. Werner and Ingbar's The Thyroid: A Fundamental and Clinical Text, 7th edn. Philadelphia: Lippincott-Raven, 1996. P.296-316.

El Ghawabi, SH; Gaafar, MA; El-Saharti, AA; Ahmed, SH; Malash, KK; Fares, R. Chronic cyanide exposure: a clinical, radioisotope, and laboratory study. *Br J Ind Med* 1975;32:215-219.

Elzubeir, EA; Davis, RH. Reduced selenium status in chicks given diets low in sulphur-containing amino acids and containing sodium nitroprusside as a source of cyanide. *Br Poult Sci* 1990;31:539-544.

Fomunyam, RT; Adegbola, AA; Oke, OL. Hydrolysis of linamarin by intestinal bacteria. *Can J Microbiol* 1984;30:1530-1531.

Frakes, RA; Sharma, RP; Wilhite, CC. Comparative metabolism of linamarin and amygdalin in hamsters. *Food Chem Toxicol* 1986;24:417-420.

Freeman, AG. Optic neuropathy and chronic cyanide intoxication: a review. *J R Soc Med* 1988;81:103-106.

Freeman, AG; Heaton, JM. The aetiology of retrolobular neuritis in Addisonian pernicious anaemia. *Lancet* 1961;1(7183):908-911.

Furbee, RB. Criminal poisoning: medical murderers. *Clin Lab Med* 2006; 26:255-273.

Gaitan, E; Cooksey, RC; Legan, J; Lindsay, RH; Ingbar, SH; Medeiros-Neto, G. Antithyroid effects in vivo and in vitro of babassu and mandioca: a staple food in goiter areas of Brazil. *Eur J Endocrinol* 1994;131:138-144.

Garlich, FM; Alsop, JA; Anderson, DL; Geller, RJ; Kalugdan, TT; Roberts, DJ; Thomas, LC. Poisoning and suicide by cyanide jewelry cleaner in the US Hmong community: A case series. *Clin Toxicol* 2012;50:136-140.

Gill, JR; Marker, E; Stajic, M. Suicide by cyanide: 17 deaths. *J Forensic Sci* 2004;49:826-828.

Grabowska, T; Skowronek, R; Nowicka, J; Sybirska, H. Prevalence of hydrogen cyanide and carboxyhaemoglobin in victims of smoke inhalation during enclosed-space fires: A combined toxicological risk. *Clin Toxicol* 2012;50:759-763.

Greer, MA; Stott, AK; Milne, KA. Effect of thiocyanate, perchlorate and other anions on thyroidal iodine metabolism. *Endocrinology* 1966;79:237-247.

Gunasekar, PG; Sun, PW; Kanthasamy, AG; Borowitz, JL; Isom, GE. Cyanide-induced neurotoxicity involves nitric oxide and reactive oxygen species generation after N-methyl-D-aspartate receptor activation. *J Pharmacol Exp Ther* 1996;277:150-155.

Gunasekar, PG; Borowitz, JL; Isom, GE. Cyanide-induced generation of oxidative species: involvement of nitric oxide synthase and cyclooxygenase-2. *J Pharmacol Exp Ther* 1998;285:236-241.

Gutzwiller, A. The effect of a diet containing cyanogenetic glycosides on the selenium status and the thyroid function of sheep. *Anim Prod* 1993;57:415-419.

Guzmán, V; Ochoa, R; Gil, A. Intoxicacion cronica por acido cianhidrico en ratas y su interaccion con la proteina y el tiosulfato de sodio de la dieta. *Revista ICA* 1977;12:241-252.

Heaton, JM; McCormick, AJA; Freeman, AG. Tobacco amblyopia: a clinical manifestation of vitamin B12 deficiency. *Lancet* 1958;2(7041):286-290.

Henny, CJ; Hallock, RJ; Hill, EE. Cyanide and migratory birds at gold mines in Nevada, USA. *Ecotoxicology* 1994:3:45-58.

Huxtable, RJ. The harmful potential of herbal and other plant products. *Drug Safety* 1990;5(suppl.1):126-136.

Ibebunjo, C; Kamalu, BP; Ihemelandu, EC. Comparison of the effects of cassava (*Manihot esculenta* Crantz), organic cyanide and inorganic cyanide on muscle and bone development in a Nigerian breed of dog. *Brit J Nutr* 1992;68:483-491.

Ivankovich, AD; Braverman, B; Kanuru, RP; Heyman, HJ; Paulissian, R. Cyanide antidotes and methods of their administration in dogs: a comparative study. *Anesthesiology* 1980;52:210-216.

Johnson, JD; Conroy, WG; Burris, KD; Isom, GE. Peroxidation of brain lipids following cyanide intoxication in mice. *Toxicology* 1987:46:21-28.

Jones DA. 1998. Why are so many food plants cyanogenic? *Phytochemistry* 47: 155–162.

Kamalu, BP. The effect of a nutritionally-balanced cassava (*Manihot esculenta* Crantz) diet on endocrine function usinga the dog as a model. 1. Pancreas. *Brit J Nutr* 1991;65:365-372.

Kamalu, BP. Pathological changes in growing dogs fed on a balanced cassava (*Manihot esculenta* Crantz) diet. *Brit J Nutr* 1993:69:921-934.

Kamalu, BP. The adverse effects of long-term cassava (*Manihot esculenta* Crantz) consumption. *Int J Food Sci Nutr* 1995;46:65-93.

Kamalu, BP; Agharanya, JC. The effect of a nutritionally-balanced cassava (*Manihot esculenta* Crantz) diet on endocrine function using the dog as a model. 2. Thyroid. *Brit J Nutr* 1991;65:373-379.

Kaneko, JJ. Thyroid function. In: Kaneko, JJ; Harvey, JW; Bruss, ML, editors. *Clinical Biochemistry of Domestic Animals, 4th ed.* San Diego: Academic Press, 2008. p.623-634.

Kanthasamy, AG; Ardelt, B; Malave, A; Mills, EM; Powley, TL; Borowitz, JL; Isom, GE. Reactive oxygen species generated by cyanide mediate toxicity in rat pheochromocytoma cells. *Toxicol Lett* 1997;93:47-54.

Katsumata, Y; Sato, K; Oya, M; Susuki, O; Yoshino, M. Kinetic analysis of the shift of aerobic anaerobic metabolism in rats during acute cyanide poisoning. *Life Sci* 1980;27:1509-1512.

Kiatsayompoo, S; Lueprasitsakul, W; Bhuripanyo, P; Graisopa, S. Diabetes mellitus in the young in Srinagarind Hospital. *J Med Assoc Thai* 1993;76:247-251.

Koenig, RJ; Brent, GA; Warne, RL; Larsen, PR; Moore, DD. Thyroid hormone receptor binds to a site in the rat growth hormone promoter required for induction by thyroid hormone. *Proc Natl Acad Sci USA* 1987;84:5670-5674.

López, JA; Martínez, FG; Martínez, RR; Horta R, JM. Variación del contenido de cianuro en Prunus brachybotrya en la segunda mitad de su desarrollo. *Veterinaria México* 1992;23:131-133.

Majak, W; Cheng, KJ. Cyanogenesis in bovine rumen fluid and pure cultures of rumen bacteria. *J Anim Sci* 1984;59:784-790.

Majak, W; McDiarmid, RE; Hall, JW; Cheng, KJ. Factors that determine rates of cyanogenesis in bovine ruminal fluid in vitro. *J Anim Sci* 1990;68:1648-1655.

Makene, MJ; Wilson, J. Biochemical studies in Tanzanian patients with ataxic tropical neuropathy. *J Neurol Neurosurg Psychiatry* 1972;35:31-33.

Maloof, F; Soodak, M. The inhibition of the metabolism of thiocyanate in the thyroid of the rat. *Endocrinology* 1959;65:106-113.

Manzano, H; Sousa, AB; Soto-Blanco, B; Guerra, JL; Maiorka, PC; Górniak, SL. Effects of long-term cyanide ingestion by pigs. *Vet Res Commun* 2007;31:93-104.

Marques, LC; Bechara, GH; Camacho, AA. Bócio parenquimatoso difuso congênito em caprinos. *Veterinária e Zootecnia* 1985;1:89-93.

Maxie, MG; Youssef, S. Nervous system. In: Gaxie, MG, editor. *Jubb, Kennedy & Palmer's Pathology of Domestic Animals, 5th ed.* Philadelphia: Saunders, 2007. p.281-457.

McCaslin, PP; Yu, XZ. Cyanide selectively augments kainate- but not NMDA-induced release of glutamate and taurine. *Eur J Pharmacol* 1992;228:73-75.

McKenzie, RA; McMicking, LI. Ataxia and urinary incontinence in cattle grazing sorghum. *Aust Vet J* 1977;53:496-497.

McMillan, DE; Geevarghese, PJ. Dietary cyanide and tropical malnutrition diabetes. *Diabetes Care* 1979;2:202-208.

Milazzo, S., Lejeune, S., Ernst, E. *Laetrile for cancer: A systematic review of the clinical evidence* (2007) Supportive Care in Cancer, 15 (6), pp. 583-595.

Milazzo, S., Ernst, E., Lejeune, S., Boehm, K., Horneber, M. Laetrile treatment for cancer. *Cochrane database of systematic reviews*, v. 11, article CD005476, 2011.

Mills, EM; Gunasekar, PG; Pavlakovic, G; Isom, GE. Cyanide-induced apoptosis and oxidative stress in differentiated PC12 cells. *J Neurochem* 1996;67:1039-1046.

Mohan, V; Mohan, R; Susheela, L; Snehalatha, C; Bharani, G; Mahajan, VK; Ramachandran, A; Viswanathan, M; Kohner, EM. Tropical pancreatic diabetes in South India: heterogeneity in clinical and biochemical profile. *Diabetologia* 1985;28:229-232.

Monekosso, GL; Annan, WGT. Clinical epidemiological observations on an ataxic syndrome in Western Nigeria. *Trop Geogr Med* 1964;4:316-323.

Moore, DGF. Retrobulbar neuritis and partial optic atrophy as sequelae of avitaminosis. *Ann Trop Med Parasitol* 1934;28:295-303.

Müller, U; Krieglstein, J. Inhibitors of lipid peroxidation protect cultured neurons against cyanide-induced injury. *Brain Res* 1995;678:265-268.

Narendranathan, M; Cheriyan, A. Lack of association between cassava consumption and tropical pancreatitis syndrome. *J Gastroenterol Hepatol* 1994;9:282-285.

Nicholson, SS. Cyanogenic plants. In: Gupta, RC, editor. *Veterinary Toxicology, 2nd edition.* London: Academic Press; 2012. p.1113-1116.

Njoh, J. Tropical ataxic neuropathy in Liberians. *Trop Geogr Med* 1990;42:92-94.

Nzwalo, H; Cliff, J. Konzo: From poverty, cassava, and cyanogen intake to toxico-nutritional neurological disease. *PLoS Negl Trop Dis* 2011;5:1051.

Odrizola, E. Poisoning by plants, mycotoxins, and algae in Argentinian livestock. In: Riet-Correa, F; Pfister, J; Schild, AL; Wieringa, TL, editors. *Poisoning by Plants, Mycotoxins and Related Toxins.* Wallington (UK): 2011. p.35-42.

Oke, O.L. The use of cassava as pig feed. *Nutr Abstr Rev Ser B* 1984;54:301-314.

Okolie, NP; Osagie, AU. Liver and kidney lesions and associated enzyme changes induced in rabbits by chronic cyanide exposure. *Food Chem Toxicol* 1999;37:745-750.

Ong, HK. Cyanogenic and goitrogenic factors in pig nutrition. *Pig News and Information* 1989;10:19-23.

Onwuka, CFI. Hydrocyanic acid contents of tropical browse and their influence on performance of goats. *Food Chem* 1992;45:5-10.

Onwuka, CFI; Akinsoyinu, AO; Tewe, OO. Role of sulphur in cyanide detoxification in ruminants. *Small Rumin Res* 1992;8:277-284.

Oruc, HH; Yilmaz, R; Bagdas, D; Ozyigit, MO. Cyanide poisoning deaths in dogs. *J Vet Med A* 2006;53:509-510.

Osuntokun, BO. Cassava diet, chronic cyanide intoxication and neuropathy in the Nigerian Africans. *World Rev Nutr Diet* 1981;36:141-73.

Osuntokun, BO; Durowoju, JE; McFarlane, H; Wilson, J. Plasma amino-acids in the Nigerian nutritional ataxic neuropathy. *Br Med J* 1968:3(5619):647-649.

Osuntokun, BO; Monekosso, GL; Wilson, J. Relationship of a degenerative tropical neuropathy to diet report of a field survey. *Br Med J* 1969;1(5643):547-550.

Osweiler, GD; Carson, TL; Buck, WB; Van Gelder, GA. Cyanide and cyanogenic plants. In: *Clinical and Diagnostic Veterinary Toxicology, 3rd edition*. Dubuque: Kendall/Hunt, 1985. p.455-459.

Owasoyo, JO; Iramain, CA. Acetylcholinesterase activity in rat brain: effect of acute cyanide intoxication. *Toxicol Lett* 1980;6:1-3.

Panigrahi, S; Rickard, J; O'Brien, GM; Gay, C. Effects of different rates of drying cassava root on its toxicity to broiler chicks. *Br Poult Sci* 1992;33:1025-1041.

Paulet, G. *L'intoxication cyanhydrique et son traitement*. Paris: Masson & Cie, 1960. 114p.

Petersen JM. 2002. Tropical pancreatitis. *J. Clin. Gastroenterol.* 35: 61–66.

Philbrick, DJ; Hopkins, JB; Hill, DC; Alexander, JC; Thomson, RG. Effects of prolonged cyanide and thiocyanate feeding in rats. *J Toxicol Environ Health* 1979;5:579-592.

Pitchumoni, CS; Jain, NK; Lowenfels, AB; DiMagno, EP. Chronic cyanide poisoning: unifying concept for alcoholic and tropical pancreatitis. *Pancreas* 1988;3:220-222.

Poulton, JE. Cyanogenic compounds in plants and their toxic effects. In: Keeler, RF; Tu, AT, editors. *Handbook of Natural Toxins - v.1 Plant and fungal toxins*. New York: Marcel Dekker, 1983. p.117-57.

Ratnakumar, JN; Rajan, A. Goitrogenic effect of cassava in broiler rabbits. *Indian J Anim Sci* 1992;62:670-676.

Richens, JE; Wesselingh, S. Fibrocalculous pancreatic diabetes in Papaua New Guinea. *Trop Geogr Med* 1988;40:84-87.

Rocha-e-Silva, RC; Cordeiro, LAV; Soto-Blanco, B. Cyanide toxicity and interference with diet selection in quail (*Coturnix coturnix*). *Comp Biochem Physiol C Toxicol Pharmacol* 2010;151:294-297.

Rodgers, GC; Condurache, CT. Antidotes and treatments for chemical warfare/terrorism agents: An evidence-based review. *Clin Pharmacol Ther* 2010;88:318-327.

Saad, AD; Camargo, VA. Intoxicação cianídrica em animais domésticos. *O Biológico* 1967;33:211-220.

Salkowski, AA; Penney, DG. Cyanide poisoning in animals and humans: a review. *Vet Human Toxicol* 1994;36:455-466.

Salkowski, AA; Penney, DG. Metabolic, cardiovascular, and neurologic aspects of acute cyanide poisoning in the rat. *Toxicol Lett* 1995;75:19-27.

Schulz, V. Clinical pharmacokinetics of nitroprusside, cyanide, thiosulphate and thiocyanate. *Clinical Pharmacokinetics* 1984;9:239-251.

Schulz, V; Gross, R; Pash, T; Busse, J; Loeschcke, G. Cyanide toxicity of sodium nitroprusside in therapeutic use with and without sodium thiosulphate. *Klinische Wochenschrift* 1982;60:1393-1400.

Scranton, JR; Nissen, WM; Halmi, NS. The kinetics of the inhibition of thyroidal iodide accumulation by thiocyanate: a reexamination. *Endocrinology* 1969;85:603-607.

Shaw, JM. Suspected cyanide poisoning in two goats caused by ingestion of crab apple leaves and fruits. *Vet Rec* 1986:119:242-243.

Smith, ADM; Duckett, S; Waters, AH. Neuropathological changes in chronic cyanide intoxication. *Nature* 1963;200:179-181.

Soto-Blanco, B; Górniak, SL. Milk transfer of cyanide and thiocyanate: cyanide exposure by lactation in goats. *Vet Res* 2003;34:213-220.

Soto-Blanco, B; Górniak, SL. Prenatal toxicity of cyanide in goats - a model for teratological studies in ruminants. *Theriogenology* 2004;62:1012-1026.

Soto-Blanco, B; Górniak, SL. Toxic effects of prolonged administration of leaves of cassava (*Manihot esculenta* Crantz) to goats. *Exp Toxicol Pathol* 2010;62:361-366.

Soto-Blanco, B; Górniak, SL; Kimura, ET. Physiopathological effects of chronic cyanide administration to growing goats - a model for cyanogenic plants ingestion. *Vet Res Commun* 2001a;25:379-389.

Soto-Blanco, B; Sousa, AB; Manzano, H; Guerra, JL; Górniak, SL. Does prolonged cyanide exposure have a diabetogenic effect? *Vet Human Toxicol* 2001b;43:106-108.

Soto-Blanco, B; Maiorka, PC; Górniak, SL. Effects of long-term low-dose cyanide administration to rats. *Ecotoxicol Environ Saf* 2002a;53:37-41.

Soto-Blanco, B; Maiorka, PC; Górniak, SL. Neuropathologic study of long term cyanide administration to goats. *Food Chem Toxicol* 2002b;40:1693-1698.

Soto-Blanco, B; Stegelmeier, BL; Górniak, SL. Clinical and pathological effects of short-term cyanide repeated dosing to goats. *J Appl Toxicol* 2005;25:445-450.

Soto-Blanco, B; Stegelmeier, BL; Pfister, JA; Gardner DR; Panter KE. Comparative effects of prolonged administration of cyanide, thiocyanate and chokecherry (*Prunus virginiana*) to goats. *J Appl Toxicol* 2008;28:356-363.

Soto-Blanco, B; Pereira, FTV; Carvalho, AF; Miglino, MA; Górniak, SL. Fetal and maternal lesions of cyanide dosing to pregnant goats. *Small Rumin Res* 2009;87:76-80.

Sousa, AB; Soto-Blanco, B; Guerra, JL; Kimura, ET; Górniak, SL. Does prolonged oral exposure to cyanide promote hepatotoxicity and nephrotoxicity? *Toxicology* 2002;174:87-95.

Sousa, AB; Manzano, H; Soto-Blanco, B; Górniak SL. Toxicokinetics of cyanide in rats, pigs and goats after oral dosing with potassium cyanide. *Arch Toxicol* 2003;77:330-334.

Sörbo, BH. On the active group in rhodanese. *Acta Chem Scand* 1951;5:1218-1219.

Sörbo, BH. Crystalline rhodanese. II. The enzyme catalyzed reaction. *Acta Chem Scand* 1953;7:1137-1145.

St. Germain, DL; Galton, VA. The deiodinase family of selenoproteins. *Thyroid* 1997;7:655-668.

Stefanidou, M; Athanaselis, S.Toxicological aspects of fire. *Vet Hum Toxicol* 2004;46:196-199.

Stevens, KR; Gallo, M. Practical considerations in the conduct chronic toxicity studies. In: Hayes, AW, editor. *Principles and Methods of Toxicology*. New York: Raven Press, 1989. p.237-250.

Sun, P; Rane, SG; Gunasekar, PG; Borowitz, JL; Isom, GE. Modulation of the NMDA receptor by cyanide: enhancement of receptor-mediated responses. *J Pharmacol Exp Ther* 1997;280:1341-1348.

Szinicz, L. History of chemical and biological warfare agentes. *Toxicology* 2005;214:167-181.

Tewe, OO; Afolabi, AO; Grissom, FEG; Littleton, GK; Oke, OL. Effect of varying dietary cyanide levels on serum thyroxine and protein metabolites in pigs. *Nutr Rep Inter* 1984;30:1249-1253.

Tewe, OO; Maner, JH; Gomez, G. Influence of cassava diets on placental thiocyanate transfer, tissue rhodanese activity and perfomance of rats during gestation. *J Sci Food Agric* 1977;28:750-756.

Tursky, T; Sajter, V. The influence of potassium cyanide poison-ing on the γ-aminobutyric acid level in rat brain. *J Neurochem* 1962;9:519-523.

Tylleskär, T; Banea, M; Bikangi, N; Fresco, L; Persson, LÅ; Rosling, H. Epidemiological evidence from Zaire for a dietary etiology of konzo, an upper motor neuron disease. *Bull World Health Organ* 1991;69:581-589.

Tylleskär, T; Banea, M; Bikangi, N; Nahimana, G; Persson, LÅ; Rosling, H. Dietary determinants of a non-progressive spastic paraparesis (Konzo): a case-referent study in a high incidence area of Zaire. *Int J Epidemiol* 1995;24:949-956.

Vannasaeng, S; Nitiyanant, W; Vichayanrat, A. Case-control study on risk factors associated with fibrocalculous pancreatic diabetes. *Diabet Med* 1988;5:835-839.

Vetter J. Plant cyanogenic glycosides. *Toxicon* 2000;38:11-36.

Vycudilik, W; Gmeiner, G. Murder by poisoning: Successful analytical investigations of spectacular cases in Austria. *Drug Test Anal* 2009;1:177-183.

Way, JL. Cyanide intoxication and its mechanism of antagonism. *Ann Rev Pharmacol Toxicol* 1984;24:451-459.

Wilson, J. Leber's hereditary optic atrhophy: a possible defect of cyanide metabolism. *Clin Sci* 1965;29:505-515.

Winek, CL; Fusia, E; Collom, WD; Shanor, SP. Cyanide poisoning as a mode of suicide. *Forensic Sci* 1978;11:51-55.

Wollman, SH. Inhibiotin by thiocyanate of accumulation of radioiodine by thyroid gland. *Am J Physiol* 1962;203:517-524.

Yamamoto, HA; Tang HW. Effects of 2-amino-7-phosphonoheptanoic acid, melatonin or NG-nitro-L-arginine on cyanide or N-methyl-D-aspartate-induced neurotoxicity in rat cortical cells. *Toxicol Lett* 1998;94:13-18.

Yang, CW; Rathinavelu, A; Borowitz, JL; Isom, GE. Activation of a calcium- and pH-dependent phospholipase A2 by cyanide in PC12 cells. *Toxicol Appl Pharmacol* 1994;124:262-267.

Youso, SL; Rockwood, GA; Logue, BA. The analysis of protein-bound thiocyanate in plasma of smokers and non-smokers as a marker of cyanide exposure. *J Anal Toxicol* 2012;36:265-269.

In: Cyanide
Editor: Benito Soto-Blanco

ISBN: 978-1-62618-297-4

Chapter 3

ESTIMATING THE HYDROGEN CYANIDE GENERATION: THERMODYNAMICS AND MASS TRANSFER

Humberto Estay *
Arcadis Chile, Santiago, Chile
Laboratory of Membrane Separation Processes (LabProSeM), Department of Chemical Engineering, University of Santiago de Chile (USACH), Santiago, Chile

ABSTRACT

The industries related to the production or use of cyanide must ensure high safety standards in order to minimize the risk to personnel exposed to hydrogen cyanide (HCN). This can be reached by accomplishing a global search of all parameters involved in the process, taking also into account the local regulations for HCN emanations. In this scenario, there is a high interest in developing methods capable of quantifying the HCN generation in different processes or equipment and in that way the implementation of remediation actions in the process operations or in the design of future projects can be taken. Nowadays, the most used method to estimate HCN generation is based on the dissociation curve of free cyanide and the Henry's law constant.

* Corresponding author: Tel +56(2) 2386 20 54, Fax +56(2) 2381 6001, E-mail: humberto.estay@arcadis.cl, humberto.estay@gmail.com.

However, this method consistently overestimates the volatilized HCN in exit gases due to there is no inclusion of the chemical interactions of cyanide with others species (e.g., zinc, copper, and nickel), and also does not consider the mass transfer of HCN, the most influential factor on HCN volatilization. The mass transfer of HCN in the liquid phase represents the main resistance of HCN transport into the gas phase, which is dependent on system characteristics such as geometry, hydrodynamics and state conditions. With this background in mind, a phenomenological method to estimate HCN generation in any system is proposed in the current chapter. This theoretical method is mainly based on the thermodynamic equilibrium of the different cyanide complexes species present in a solution, the phase equilibrium behaviour based on the Henry's law equilibrium, and the mass transfer of HCN into the air based on a resistances-in-series model to determine the HCN content in the liquid and gas phases. In addition, the proposed method also evaluates the effect of system conditions (temperature, pressure, and pH) and the operation characteristics or equipment used. Thus, this phenomenological method can be a powerful and valuable tool for quantifying HCN generation in realistic simulations, along with providing rapid identification of risk conditions in the process and more criteria for investment project decision making.

NOMENCLATURE

α	Mass transfer correlation parameter, dimensionless
β	Product of equilibrium constant, dimensionless
ε	Porosity, dimensionless
$\varepsilon_{A,B}$	Lennard-Jones energy parameter, K
ϕ	Packing fraction , dimensionless
μ	Viscosity, kg/m s
ρ	Density, kg/m^3
σ	Lennard-Jones collision diameter, Å
τ	Fiber tortuosity, dimensionless
χ	Mass transfer correlation parameter, dimensionless
Φ	Solvent association factor, dimensionless
Ω	Lennard-Jones collision integral for diffusion, dimensionless
a	Specific area (mass transfer area per equipment volume), m^2/m^3
A	Area, m^2
C	Molar concentration, mol/m^3
d	Diameter, m
D	Diffusion coefficient, m^2/s
e	Fiber thickness, m
F	Feed solution flow, m^3/s

g	Gravity, m/s^2
Gz	Graetz number, dimensionless
h	Standard enthalpy, J/mol
H	Henry's law constant, Pa/mol fraction
J	HCN molar flux, $mol/(m^2 s)$
k	Local mass transfer coefficient, m/s
K_i	Equilibrium constant of the i-th specie, dimensionless
K	Overall mass transfer coefficient, m/s
L	Characteristic length, m
m	Partition coefficient, dimensionless
M	Metal, dimensionless
$M_{A,B}$	Molecular weight, g/mol
n	Number of fibers, dimensionless
N	Overall transfer rate, mol/s
pK_a	Logarithmic exponent of dissociation constant, dimensionless
P	Pressure, Pa
R	Universal gas constant, J/(molK)
R_0	Radius of the spherical solute in Equation 48, m
Re	Reynolds number, dimensionless
Sc	Schmidt number, dimensionless
Sh	Sherwood number, dimensionless
T	Temperature, K
v	Velocity, m/s
V_A	Molar volume of the solute at its normal boiling point, cm^3/mol
V	Tank volume, m^3
W/V	Power-tank volume ratio, W/m^3
x	Mol fraction in the liquid phase, dimensionless
y	Mol fraction in the gas phase, dimensionless
z	Boundary layer in a phase for natural convection

Subscripts

1	Referred to the equipment end
2	Referred to the equipment end
a	Referred to thermodynamic equilibrium
A	Referred to specie A
B	Referred to specie B
AB	Referred to the interaction of species A and B
cation	Referred to metal cation
C	Referred to the characteristic length
g	Referred to the gas phase
h	Referred to the hydraulic diameter
HCN	Referred to HCN

HCN0	Referred to the initial HCN concentration
HCNL	Referred to the HCN content in the liquid phase
HCNg	Referred to the HCN content in the gas phase
HCNLinlet	Referred to HCN concentration at inlet of equipment
HCNLoutlet	Referred to HCN concentration at outlet of equipment
HCNLt	Referred to HCN concentration at time t
HCN-air	Referred to the HCN diffusion in the air phase
HCN-liquid	Referred to the HCN diffusion in the liquid phase
HCN-P	Referred to the HCN diffusion in the P phase
i	Referred to i-specie
in	Referred to internal diameter
j	Referred to the cyanide mol in a metal-cyanide specie
Liquid	Referred to the liquid phase
L	Referred to the liquid phase
m	Referred to the metal
ml	Referred to the logarithmic mean driving force
out	Referred to external diameter
p	Referred to pore size
P	Referred to the phase
T	Referred to the total element content

Superscripts

*	Referred to the pseudo-equilibrium interface
0	Referred to superficial velocity
g	Referred to gas phase
HCN	Referred to HCN
j	Referred to the cyanide mol in a metal-cyanide specie
L	Referred to liquid phase
o	Referred to the interface

1. Introduction

In the last years the industrial processes working with cyanide, such as electroplating, insecticides production, gold and silver mining, cosmetic industry, among others, are subjected to more stringent regulations with regard to environmental and the workplace safety (Longsdon, Hagelstein & Mudder, 1999; Mudder & Botz, 2004), and process optimization by reduction of operational costs (Fleming, 2005). In this context, equipment design and plant operation must consider this approach to ensure the safety of the personnel and minimize cyanide losses.

The cyanide is a toxic reagent, causing tissue hypoxia and "cyanosis" in humans exposed to cyanide by inhalation, ingestion or absorption through the skin. The most toxic form of cyanide is the hydrogen cyanide (HCN), leading to death in minutes at concentrations above 250 ppm in air (Longsdon, Hagelstein & Mudder, 1999). For this reason, the current operations measure HCN emanations using gas sensors and alarms set at specific values, thereby avoiding risk to human health. On this regard, local regulations have limited the HCN concentration at 4.7 ppm for worker exposure, as well as the cyanidation processes operating in conditions of pH higher than 10.5, which minimize HCN content in their solutions. Overall these actions have allowed the establishment of safer operational conditions for personnel, although do not predict or quantify the HCN emanations or control risk conditions, which it could limit the current operational actions (except the operation at higher pH). Additionally, in the last years the cyanide users are focused on the incorporation of cyanide recovery processes to reduce cyanide consumptions (Fleming, 2005). These processes are based on the decrease of pH lower than 7, maximizing the HCN content in solution and increasing the risk of HCN emanations. In this context, the equipment design for these processes must include parameters or additional unit operations that minimize and avoid the HCN gas generation (Estay et al., 2012).

Summing up, the estimation of HCN generation is a relevant issue to predict the risk of certain unit operations in a process and the design aspects which are necessary to include in the first stages of a project. The most simple and widely used method to estimate HCN emanation is based on the Henry's law applied to the cyanide concentration in solution (Dzombak, Ghosh and Young, 2006), neglecting the effect of the mass transfer resistances, which it causes an overestimation of HCN gas generation. Nowadays, few studies have included the effect of the mass transfer resistances on the HCN gas generation (Young, Zhao and Theis, 2006; Lotter, 2006; Estay et al., 2012), many of which have been applied to specific systems and using different assumptions to estimate physical properties and metals content effect in solution.

A general method to estimate and characterize the HCN gas generation in diverse systems is presented in this study, which unifies the thermodynamic of metal-cyanide complexes in the solution in order to estimate the dissolved HCN content, the Henry's law to describe the phase equilibrium between the solution and the air, and the mass transfer mechanism in the solution and in the air.

2. Thermodynamics of Aqueous Cyanide Species

2.1. Aqueous Forms of Cyanide

Cyanide forms simple salts which dissolve and ionize in water forming their respective metal cation and free cyanide ions (Marsden and House, 2006), as follows:

$$MCN \longleftrightarrow M^{+} + CN^{-} \tag{1}$$

Likewise, cyanide ions hydrolyze in water forming HCN and hydroxyl (OH^-) ions, increasing the pH, as shown in Equation (2). HCN is a weak acid, which incompletely dissociates in water according to Equation (3), (Marsden and House, 2006).

$$CN^{-} + H_2O \longleftrightarrow HCN + OH^{-} \tag{2}$$

$$HCN \longleftrightarrow H^{+} + CN^{-} \tag{3}$$

The logarithmic exponent of the dissociation constant pK_a of HCN at 25ºC is 9.21 (Izzat et al., 1962; Lu et al., 2002). pH values higher than 9.21 increase the cyanide anion content in comparison with the dissolved HCN content while pH values lower than 9.21 promote the presence of dissolved HCN in solution. A typical curve of HCN distribution in aqueous solution at 25ºC is shown in Figure 1. Thus, the amount of HCN in solution depends on the system pH (Estay et al, 2012).

The Equation (3) represents the free cyanide species for cyanide, dissolved HCN and soluble cyanide anion (CN^-). The free cyanide anion CN^- can generate complexes with other many metals species, such as copper, zinc, nickel, cadmium among others, which vary widely in stability and solubility (Marsden and House, 2006).

$$M^{+x} + jCN^{-} \longleftrightarrow M(CN)_j^{-(j-x)} \tag{4}$$

The metal-cyanide species can be classified into two categories, weak acid dissociable (WAD) and strong cyanide complexes (SAD), according to the strength of the bonding between the metal and the cyanide ion. The classification of the different cyanide species is based on the equilibrium constant value (Marsden and House, 2006) or the acidic conditions needed to dissociate (Gosh, Dzombak and Wong-Chong, 2006). Both criteria can be taken to establish a classification, although the effect of pH and concentration of the cyanide-species in solution determine the stability of these complexes under specific conditions. Thereby, cyanide species contents in solution can be determined at a fixed temperature by the equilibrium constant (K_i) described by Equation (5):

$$K_i = \frac{[M^{+x}][CN^-]^j}{[M(CN)_j^{-(j-x)}]} \tag{5}$$

A brief list of the most important aqueous cyanide species, classified as free, WAD or SAD cyanide is shown in Table 1. Other species such as cyanate, thiocyanate, and metal-thiocyanate complexes can be also considered.

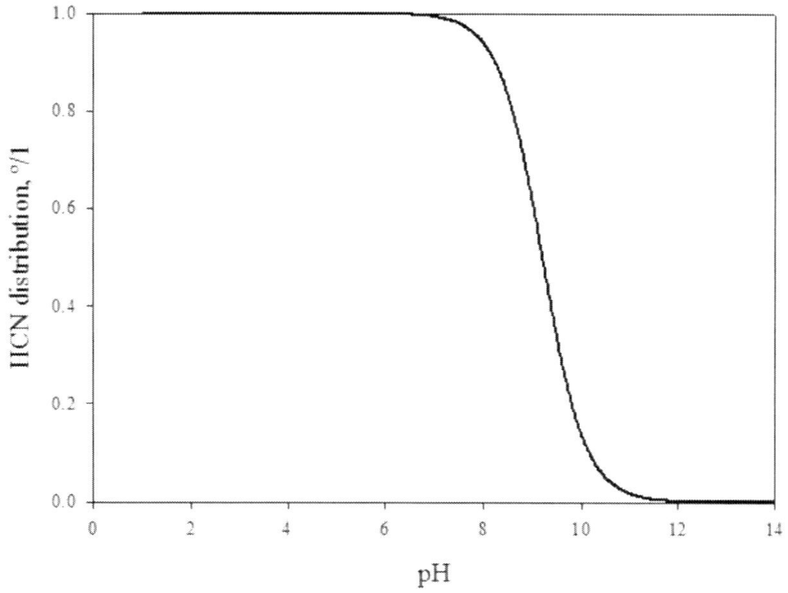

Figure 1. HCN distribution in aqueous solution at 25°C.

Table 1. Aqueous cyanide species classified according to stability.

Classification criterion	Cyanide species
Free cyanide	CN^-, HCN
WAD	$Cd(CN)_2$, $Cd(CN)_3^-$, $Cd(CN)_4^{-2}$, $Zn(CN)_2$, $Zn(CN)_3^-$, $Zn(CN)_4^{-2}$, $Zn(CN)_5^{-3}$, $Ag(CN)_2^-$, $Ag(CN)_3^{-2}$, $Cu(CN)_2^-$, $Cu(CN)_3^{-2}$, $Cu(CN)_4^{-3}$, $Ni(CN)_3^-$, $Ni(CN)_4^{-2}$, $HgCN^+$, $Hg(CN)_2$, $Hg(CN)_3^-$, $Hg(CN)_4^{-2}$
SAD	$Fe(CN)_6^{-3}$, $Fe(CN)_6^{-4}$, $Au(CN)_2^-$, $Au(CN)_4^-$, $Co(CN)_6^{-3}$, $Co(CN)_6^{-4}$, $Pt(CN)_4^{-2}$

2.2. Thermodynamic Behaviour of Aqueous Metal-Cyanide Species

As described earlier, the metal-cyanide complexes can be classified based on their stability, which depends on pH and concentration of each compound in solution, meaning activity. Thus, a cyanidation system can be characterized by pH and the equilibrium constants of each cyanide species present in a solution (Equation 5). It is known that the equilibrium constant is affected by temperature, and its relationship is described by the van't Hoff equation as follows (Marsden et al., 2006).

$$\frac{dLnK_i}{dT} = \frac{\Delta h_i}{RT^2} \tag{6}$$

In the above equation Δh_i is the standard enthalpy change of each reaction, R is the universal gas constant (8.314 J/mol K) and the subscript i indicates the corresponding equilibrium constant described earlier. The values of Δh_i and K_i for common equilibrium relationships are presented in the Table 2. Additional Δh_i and K_i values can be found in literature (Xue and Osseo-Asare, 1985; Senanayake, 2008). On the other hand, it is possible to make elemental mass balances for each cyanide species, which can be represented by Equations (7) and (8).

$$[CN]_T = [CN^-] + [HCN] + \sum_m \sum_j j[M_m(CN)_j] \tag{7}$$

Table 2. Values of equilibrium constants and standard enthalpy change for common cyanide species.

Equation	$K_i$at 25°C	ΔH_i at 25°C, KJ/mol	Source
$HCN \longleftrightarrow H^+ + CN^-$	$6.17\ 10^{-10}$	43.5	(Izzat et al., 1962)
$Cd^{+2} + 2CN^- \longleftrightarrow Cd(CN)_2^0$	$1.32 \cdot 10^{11}$	-	(Marsden and House, 2006)
$Cd(CN)_2^0 + CN^- \longleftrightarrow Cd(CN)_3^-$	$3.39 \cdot 10^5$	-	(Marsden and House, 2006)
$Cd(CN)_3^- + CN^- \longleftrightarrow Cd(CN)_4^{-2}$	$1.86 \cdot 10^1$	-	(Marsden and House, 2006)
$Zn^{+2} + 2CN^- \longleftrightarrow Zn(CN)_2^0$	$1.17 \cdot 10^{11}$	-63.2	(Izzat et al., 1965)
$Zn(CN)_2^0 + CN^- \longleftrightarrow Zn(CN)_3^-$	$9.55 \cdot 10^4$	-28.5	(Izzat et al., 1965)
$Zn(CN)_3^- + CN^- \longleftrightarrow Zn(CN)_4^{-2}$	$3.72\ 10^3$	-20.4	(Izzat et al., 1965)
$Ag^+ + CN^- \longleftrightarrow AgCN(s)$	$4.57 \cdot 10^{15}$	-	(Marsden and House, 2006)
$Ag^+ + 2CN^- \longleftrightarrow Ag(CN)_2^-$	$2.75 \cdot 10^{20}$	-137.7	(Izzat et al., 1967)
$Ag(CN)_2^- + CN^- \longleftrightarrow Ag(CN)_3^{-2}$	$3.55 \cdot 10^1$	-2.5	(Izzat et al., 1967)
$Cu^+ + CN^- \longleftrightarrow CuCN(s)$	$1.0\ 10^{20}$	128	(Lu et al., 2002)
$CuCN + CN^- \longleftrightarrow Cu(CN)_2^-$	$8.71\ 10^3$	-121.8	(Izzat et al., 1967)
$Cu(CN)_2^- + CN^- \longleftrightarrow Cu(CN)_3^{-2}$	$2.0\ 10^5$	-46.5	(Izzat et al., 1967)
$Cu(CN)_3^{-2} + CN^- \longleftrightarrow Cu(CN)_4^{-3}$	$3.16\ 10^1$	-46.9	(Izzat et al., 1967)
$Ni^{+2} + 4CN^- \longleftrightarrow Ni(CN)_4^{-2}$	$1.26 \cdot 10^{30}$	-183.6	(Christensen et al., 1963)
$Hg^{+2} + CN^- \longleftrightarrow HgCN^+$	$1.0 \cdot 10^{17}$	-96.3	(Christensen et al., 1965)
$HgCN^+ + CN^- \longleftrightarrow Hg(CN)_2^0$	$5.62 \cdot 10^{15}$	-106.8	(Christensen et al., 1965)
$Hg(CN)_2^0 + CN^- \longleftrightarrow Hg(CN)_3^-$	$3.63 \cdot 10^3$	-31.8	(Christensen et al., 1965)
$Hg(CN)_3^- + CN^- \longleftrightarrow Hg(CN)_4^{-2}$	$4.57 \cdot 10^2$	-30.1	(Christensen et al., 1965)
$Fe^{+3} + 6CN^- \longleftrightarrow Fe(CN)_6^{-3}$	$3.98 \cdot 10^{43}$	-293.7	(Watt et al., 1965)
$Fe^{+2} + 6CN^- \longleftrightarrow Fe(CN)_6^{-4}$	$2.51 \cdot 10^{35}$	-359.1	(Watt et al., 1965)
$Au^+ + CN^- \longleftrightarrow AuCN(s)$	$6.04 \cdot 10^{32}$	-	(Adams and Fleming, 1989)
$Au^+ + 2CN^- \longleftrightarrow Au(CN)_2^-$	$2.0 \cdot 10^{39}$	-	(Marsden and House, 2006)
$Co^{+3} + 6CN^- \longleftrightarrow Co(CN)_6^{-3}$	$1.0 \cdot 10^{64}$	-	(Marsden and House, 2006)
$Co^{+2} + 6CN^- \longleftrightarrow Co(CN)_6^{-4}$	$1.26 \cdot 10^{19}$	-	(Marsden and House, 2006)

$$[M_m]_T = [M_{cation}] + \sum_j [M_m(CN)_j] \tag{8}$$

Where, T represents the total compound presents as different specie, m represents the metal m and j represents the complex j of the metal m, associated to the cyanide mol numbers. Thus, the quantity of equations will be determined by the quantity of metals present in the solution. For example, a solution containing cyanide, copper and nickel will be represented by three equations:

$$\begin{aligned}[CN]_T &= [CN^-] + [HCN] + [CuCN] + 2[Cu(CN)_2^-] + 3[Cu(CN)_3^{-2}] \\ &+ 4[Cu(CN)_4^{-3}] + 4[Ni(CN)_4^{-2}]\end{aligned} \tag{9}$$

$$[Cu]_T = [Cu^+] + [CuCN] + [Cu(CN)_2^-] + [Cu(CN)_3^{-2}] + [Cu(CN)_4^{-3}] \tag{10}$$

$$[Ni]_T = [Ni^{+2}] + [Ni(CN)_4^{-2}] \tag{11}$$

Besides, a general equation can be obtained to characterize each cyanidation system, as function of pH, temperature and species concentrations, solving simultaneously Equations (5-8).

$$[CN_T] = [CN^-]\left[1 + \frac{10^{-pH}}{10^{-pK_a}}\right] + \sum_m [M_m] \frac{\sum_j j\beta_{mj}[CN^-]^j}{1 + \sum_j \beta_{mj}[CN^-]^j} \tag{12}$$

Where β_{mj} is the product of the K_i values of each metal-cyanide complex j for the metal m, as shown Equation (13).

$$\beta_{mj} = K_{m1} \cdot K_{m2} \cdots K_{mn} \tag{13}$$

In this last equation the subscript j is conditioned to the cyanide mol contained in the metal-cyanide complex. Then, Equations (12) and (13) can be solved for the example developed for cyanide, copper and nickel exposed earlier (Equations 9-11):

$$[CN_T] = [CN^-]\left[1 + \frac{10^{-pH}}{10^{-pK_a}}\right] +$$
$$[Cu]\frac{\left[\beta_{Cu1}[CN^-] + 2\beta_{Cu2}[CN^-]^2 + 3\beta_{Cu3}[CN^-]^3 + 4\beta_{Cu4}[CN^-]^4\right]}{\left[1 + \beta_{Cu1}[CN^-] + \beta_{Cu2}[CN^-]^2 + \beta_{Cu3}[CN^-]^3 + \beta_{Cu4}[CN^-]^4\right]} +$$
$$[Ni]\frac{\beta_{Ni4}[CN^-]^4}{1 + \beta_{Ni4}[CN^-]^4} \tag{14}$$

$$\beta_{Cuj} = K_{Cu1} \cdot K_{Cu2} \cdots K_{Cuj}$$
$$\beta_{Ni4} = K_{Ni4} \tag{15}$$

These equations are very useful to determine the behaviour of metal-cyanides species and pH, therefore the HCN contained in the solution that could be generated by a process.

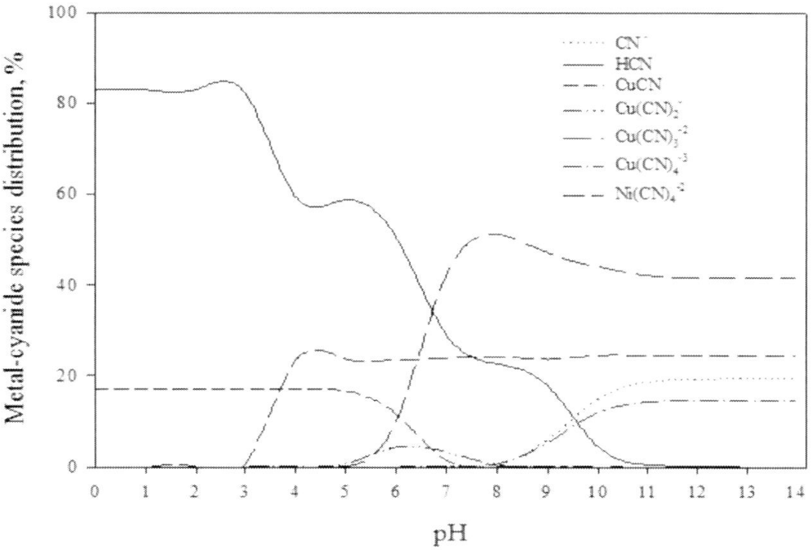

Figure 2. Distribution of cyanides species for a system containing 250 mg/L Cu, 80 mg/L Ni and 600 mg/L total cyanide at 15°C.

From the equations above-mentioned, the distribution of the cyanide species for diverse systems can be obtained. Figure 2 shows diverse distribution curves for a system containing 600 mg/L total cyanide, 250 mg/L copper and 80 mg/L nickel at 15ºC.

2.3. Liquid-Gas Phase Equilibrium of Hydrogen Cyanide

The HCN contained in a solution generates a liquid-gas interface, where the dissolved HCN is volatilized into the air phase as gaseous HCN. At the interface, the equal chemical potentials between both phases generate a liquid-gas phase equilibrium which can be described by Henry's law for HCN (Smith et al., 2005).

$$P\, y_{HCN} = H_{HCN}\, x_{HCN} \tag{16}$$

Here, P is the pressure of the system (atm), y_{HCN} is the mol fraction of HCN in the gas phase, H_{HCN} is the Henry's law constant (atm/mol fraction) and x_{HCN} is the mol fraction of HCN in the liquid phase. The Henry's law constant depends on temperature in a logarithmic relationship. Different models have been used to study the dependence of temperature on the Henry's law constant. A recent research study conducted by Ma and co-workers (2010) presented an interesting compilation and comparison of Henry's law constant values and equations from different sources and proposed a new model to determine the Henry's law constant for low cyanide concentrations and a limited temperatures range (287-311 K) (Ma et al., 2010). Furthermore, a meaningful model for a wider temperatures range (Bodek et al., 1988) has been previously cited. In turn, an empirical equation was recently reported by Estay and co-workers (2012) which is based on experimental data. All these models are very useful for determining HCN concentrations and temperatures ranges more usual in the industry. These three models are shown in Table 3, as originally reported, and Figure 3 presents the results for each model depending on temperature.

The models included in Table 3 estimate similar Henry's law constant values for low temperatures (<25°C). However, the curve estimated by the Ma and co-workers model overestimates the expected values for temperatures higher than 30°C, whilethe models developed by Bodek et al. (1988) and Estay et al. (2012) present a similar tendency, even extrapolating outside the original experimental temperature range. In this sense, these last two models can be applied in a wide temperature range, although the model proposed by Estay et al. (2012) also works for a wide HCN concentration range.

Table 3. Different models for Henry's law constant depending on temperature.

Model	Units	Valid range	H_{HCN} at 20°C, atm/mol fraction	Source	Equation
$\log H_{HCN} = -\frac{1279.9}{T} + 6.238$	T(K) H_{HCN}(mmHg/M)	20-95°C 180-9,000 mg/L	5.75	Bodek et al., 1988	17
$\ln H_{HCN} = \frac{8205.7}{T} - 25.323$	T(K) H_{HCN}(M/atm)	14-38°C 0.8-36 mg/L	3.85	Ma et al., 2010	18
$\ln H_{HCN} = -\frac{3638.8}{T} + 18.539$	T(K) H_{HCN}(kPa/mol fraction)	0-50°C 0-35,000 mg/L	4.52	Estay et al., 2012	19

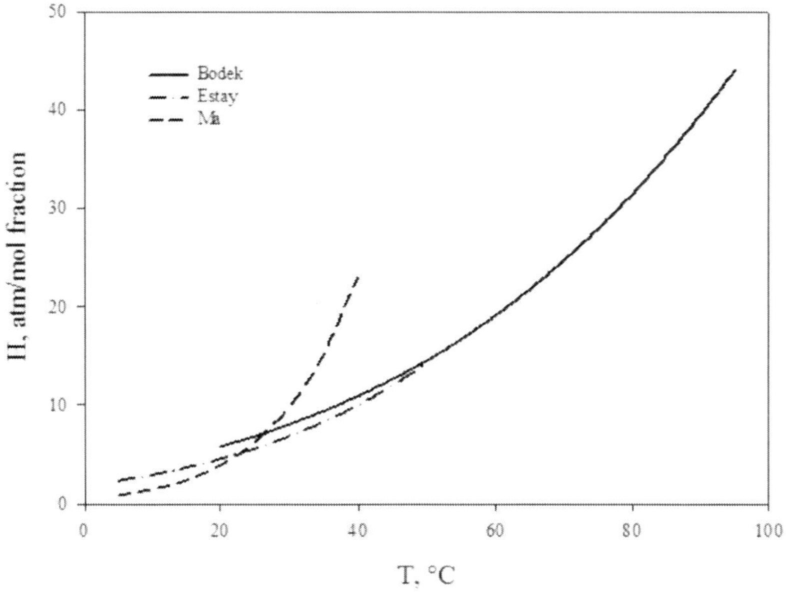

Figure 3. Henry's law constant curves from models reported earlier.

For processes operating at typical operational conditions, the Henry's law constant ranges from 2 to 7 atm/mol fraction, values 100-times lower than those found for other gases such as H_2S (Perry and Green, 1997). This fact is relevant for industrial processes, since the HCN contained in the liquid phase tends to remain in solution, inhibiting rapid HCN volatilization. However, the estimation of HCN gas generation by thermodynamic phase equilibrium is valid for static systems where the chemical potentials in both phases are equals. For dynamic systems, like the typical industrial processes, the chemical potentials are not equal in the bulk phases, but only at the liquid-gas interface. Thus, HCN transfer from the bulk of the liquid phase into the gas phase is determined by the kinetics of mass transfer.

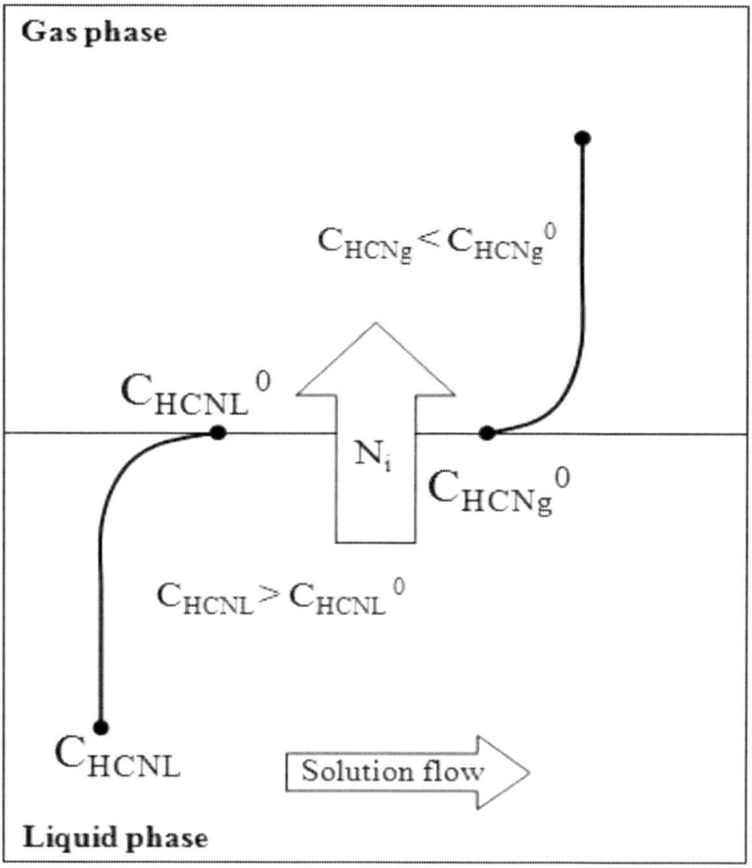

Figure 4. Schematic mechanism of the HCN mass transfer from the bulk of the liquid phase into the bulk of the gas phase (Estay et al., 2012).

3. Mass Transfer of Hydrogen Cyanide

Mass transfer of HCN from cyanide solution into the air is determined by the difference of chemical potentials between liquid phase and gas phase (Bird et al., 2007, Cussler, 2009). The HCN transfer rate for this system can be estimated by a HCN concentration gradient between the bulk and the interface in the liquid phase, and a mass transfer coefficient, which is dependent on the system geometry, physical properties of fluids and operational conditions (Cussler, 2009; Treybal, 1980). Thus, the HCN transfer rate can be described by:

$$J_{HCN} = k_L (C_{HCNL} - C^o_{HCNL}) \tag{20}$$

Here, J_{HCN} is the HCN molar flux per transfer area (mol/m^{2}s), k_L the local mass transfer coefficient of liquid phase (m/s), C^o_{HCNL} the concentration of HCN in equilibrium at the interface of liquid phase (mol/m^3), and C_{HCNL} the concentration of HCN in the bulk of liquid phase (mol/m^3). Equation (20) could be rewritten based on the gas phase, in such a way that the magnitude of the HCN transfer rate would be similar to the one described when using the liquid phase (Treybal, 1980). Figure 4 shows a schematic diagram for the HCN mass transfer promoted by a concentration gradient from the bulk of the liquid phase to the bulk of the gas phase, HCN being volatilized at the interface.

3.1. Resistances-in-Series Mass Transfer Model

The earlier description of HCN mass transfer represents only local profiles. However, an overall analysis should be made for continuous systems such as an industrial process. The overall HCN transfer rate is specified by the concentration profiles in the volume of each equipment studied. Thus, to quantify the overall HCN transfer rate in the system, it is necessary to solve Equation (20) for each equipment applying an infinitesimal mass balance. Treybal (1980) developed these expressions and proposed the following general equation:

$$N_{HCN} = K_L A \, \Delta C^L_{ml} \tag{21}$$

Here N_{HCN} is the overall HCN transfer rate (mol/s) transferred from cyanide solution into the air, K_L is the overall mass transfer coefficient based on liquid phase (m/s), A is the total mass transfer area (m^2), and ΔC_{ml}^L is the logarithmic mean driving force in the liquid phase (mol/m^3) (Bird et al., 2007; Treybal, 1980) expressed by:

$$\Delta C_{ml}^{L} = \frac{\left(C_{HCNL} - C^{*}_{HCNL}\right)_1 - \left(C_{HCNL} - C^{*}_{HCNL}\right)_2}{\ln\left[\frac{\left(C_{HCNL} - C^{*}_{HCNL}\right)_1}{\left(C_{HCNL} - C^{*}_{HCNL}\right)_2}\right]} \tag{22}$$

Where 1 and 2 represent the equipment input/output conditions, C_{HCNL} is the concentration of HCN in the bulk of the liquid phase (mol/m^3) and C_{HCNL}^* is the pseudo-equilibrium concentration of HCN in the liquid phase, represented by a partition constant as follows:

$$C^{*}_{HCNL} = C_L \frac{y_{HCN}}{m_{HCN}} \tag{23}$$

Here C_L is the total concentration of the liquid phase (mol/m^3), y_{HCN} is the concentration of HCN in the bulk of the air (mol fraction) and m_{HCN} is the partition constant (H_{HCN}/P) in mol of HCN in the gas phase per mol of HCN in the liquid phase.

The pseudo-equilibrium concentration mentioned here is useful to incorporate the overall mass transfer coefficient in the estimate of the transferred solute flow. The overall mass transfer coefficients are widely used to quantify the mass transfer of solutes by the incorporation of the mass transfer resistance concept (Cussler, 2009; Treybal, 1980). For cyanidation systems, the volatilization of HCN is controlled by the mass transfer resistance in the liquid and gas phases (Estay et al., 2012), which it can be estimated by using a mass transfer model of resistances-in-series based on the liquid phase expressed by:

$$\frac{1}{K_L} = \frac{1}{k_L} + \frac{1}{m_{HCN} k_g} \tag{24}$$

Where k_L is the local mass transfer coefficient in the liquid phase and k_g is the local mass transfer coefficient in the gas phase. The overall mass transfer resistance in an industrial process is represented by the term $1/K_L$, while the local mass transfer resistances in the gas and liquid phases are described by $1/k_g$ and $1/k_L$, respectively. The resistances-in-series mass transfer model is based on one-phase diffusion (i.e. liquid phase) and assumes that the overall mass transfer resistance only occurs in this phase. Thus, the phase equilibrium at the interface can be especified by using the bulk concentration of the other phase (i.e. gas phase) in equilibrium with the pseudo-equilibrium concentration. A schematic model of the process using pseudo-equilibrium concentrations is depicted in Figure 5. On the other hand, when the resistances-in-series model is based on the gas phase, the Equations 21-24 can be rewrite as shown below:

$$N_{HCN} = K_g A \, \Delta C_{ml}^g \tag{21a}$$

$$\Delta C_{ml}^g = \frac{\left(C_{HCNg}^* - C_{HCNg}\right)_1 - \left(C_{HCNg}^* - C_{HCNg}\right)_2}{\ln\left[\frac{\left(C_{HCNg}^* - C_{HCNg}\right)_1}{\left(C_{HCNg}^* - C_{HCNg}\right)_2}\right]} \tag{22a}$$

$$C_{HCNg}^* = C_g m_{HCN} x_{HCN} \tag{23a}$$

$$\frac{1}{K_g} = \frac{m_{HCN}}{k_L} + \frac{1}{k_g} \tag{24a}$$

Where K_g is the overall mass transfer coefficient based on gas phase (m/s), ΔC_{ml}^g is the logarithmic mean driving force in the gas phase (mol/m^3), C_{HCNg}^* is the pseudo-equilibrium concentration of HCN in the gas phase, and C_g is the total concentration of the gas phase that can be estimated by the ideal gas law for low pressures.

The resistances-in-series mass transfer model is useful for industrial processes where the determination of concentrations at the interface is complex. This model has been applied for different separation or volatilization processes such as gas absorption in packed towers (Treybal, 1980), supercritical separation of fluids in membrane contactors (Estay et al., 2007),

HCN volatilization in the SART process (Estay et al., 2012), and HCN volatilization in tailings (Lotter, 2006), having a good performance for design, prediction or validation.

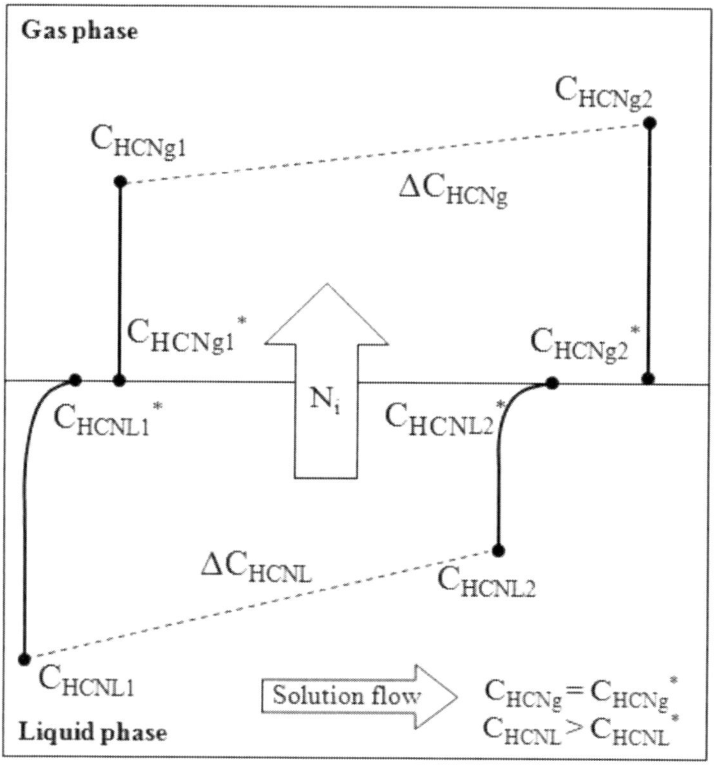

Figure 5. Schematic mechanism of the gaseous HCN generation in an equipment of an industrial process. Subscripts 1 and 2 correspond to the ends of the equipment (Estay et al., 2012).

3.2. Mass Transfer Correlations for Different Systems

The estimation of the local mass transfer coefficients is based on the Chilton-Colburn's correlations (Bird et al., 2007; Cussler, 2009), which consider the system geometry and the following dimensionless numbers: Reynolds (*Re*), Schmidt (*Sc*) and Sherwood (*Sh*). The local mass transfer coefficient in every equipment item, for both phases, can be determined by mass transfer correlations as:

$$Sh = \alpha \, \mathrm{Re}^{\chi} \, Sc^{1/3} \tag{25}$$

The parameters α and χ represent the effect of system geometry, thus determining the hydrodynamic of the equipment. Besides, *Sh*, *Re* and *Sc* numbers are defined by Equations (26-28).

$$Sh = \frac{k_P L_C}{D_{HCN-P}} \tag{26}$$

$$\mathrm{Re} = \frac{\rho_P v_P L_C}{\mu_P} \tag{27}$$

$$Sc = \frac{\mu_P}{\rho_P D_{HCN-P}} \tag{28}$$

In the above equations, the subscript *P* represents the phase involved (gas or liquid), $D_{HCN\text{-}P}$ is the diffusion coefficient of HCN in the phase *P*, L_C is the characteristic length of the equipment (e.g. diameter, length, hydraulic diameter, among others), ρ_P is the phase density, v_P is the phase flow velocity in the equipment, and μ_P is the phase viscosity.

There are different available correlations in the literature for assessment of local mass transfer coefficients. Each one of these correlations corresponds to specific system geometry. Hence, the local mass transfer coefficients for both phases can be determined according to the specific hydrodynamic of each equipment. For example, the local mass transfer coefficients for an agitated and sealed tank, with air flowing on the top of the liquid interface can be estimated by a flat plate correlation for gas phase and using an agitated tank correlation for the liquid phase. Treybal (1980) reported a mass transfer correlation for flat plate systems under laminar (Re<50,000) and turbulent (Re>50,000) flow conditions. Both correlations are shoen in Equations (29) and (30). On the other hand, mass transfer correlations for the liquid phase are strongly dependent on equipment geometry. Cussler (2009) reported a mass transfer correlation for agitated tank systems, which is related to the agitation power/tank volume ratio (*W/V*), characteristic length of the tank (L_C) and physical properties of the liquid:

$$Sh = 0.664\ \mathrm{Re}^{0.5}\ Sc^{1/3} \tag{29}$$

$$Sh = 0.023\mathrm{Re}^{0.83}\ Sc^{1/3} \tag{30}$$

$$Sh = 0.13\left[\frac{L_C^4\,(W/V)\,\rho^2}{\mu^3}\right]^{1/4} Sc^{1/3} \tag{31}$$

For static systems, such as storage tanks or thickeners where both phases (gas and liquid) are relatively quiet since the solution flow rate should be sufficiently low, the local mass transfer coefficients in the liquid and gas phases should be estimated by using a natural convection model (Treybal, 1980):

$$k_P = \frac{D_{HCN-P}}{z} \tag{32}$$

Where, z is the distance between the bulk and interface of phases (the boundary layer). These correlations (Equations 29-32) were applied in a previous research (Estay et al., 2012) to estimate the HCN gas generation in a cyanide recovery process namely SART (Sulphidization, Acidification, Recycling and Thickening). This process comprises the following equipment units: agitated and sealed reactors, tanks and thickeners at different pH conditions. The aim of that work was estimate risk conditions of the process and design values for the scrubbing system, which removes the HCN gas generated.

In terms of equipment design for cyanide recovery, such as desorption and absorption packed towers for AVR (Acidification, Volatilization and Regeneration) process (Smith and Mudder, 1991) or membranes contactors for GFMA process (Estay et al., 2013; Estay et al., 2011), there are useful correlations to characterize the HCN mass transport. The mass transfer correlations for absorption and desorption processes in packed towers depend on the type of packing (e.g. rashing rings, pall rings, berl saddles, among others). Correlations for packed towers have been reported by different authors (Treybal, 1980; McCabe et al., 2004; Geankopolis, 1993; Cussler, 2009), although the support of the packing suppliers should be considered for a specific feed solution. Equation (33) shows a correlation reported by Cussler (2009).

$$\frac{k_P}{v^0} = 1.17\left(\frac{d_p v^0 \rho}{\mu}\right)^{-0.42}\left(\frac{\mu}{\rho D_{HCN^{-}-P}}\right)^{-0.67} \quad (33)$$

Here, d_p is the particle diameter (reported by supplier or estimated by Equation (34) and v_0 is the superficial velocity (velocity without packing).

$$d_p = \frac{6(1-\varepsilon)}{a} \quad (34)$$

Where, ε is the porosity of the particle, and a is the specific area (mass transfer area per packing volume). The design of packed towers must also include the estimation of pressure drop in the packing in order to adequately estimate the fan power.

On the other hand, the membranes contactors depend on configuration of the module (inlet and outlet flows, baffles orientation and length of the module). There are many correlations in the literature that aim to establish equations for membrane contactors, for the shell and lumen side, (Gabelman and Hwang, 1999; Shen et al., 2010); hence the selection of the more accurate correlation will depend on the adjustment to experimental or industrial results. For the lumen side, the Lévêque correlation has been proposed under laminar flow conditions when Graetz number (Gz) is higher than 6 (Shen et al., 2010), as shown Equation (35). For Gz numbers lower than 6, the Equation (36) is proposed (Shen et al., 2010).

$$Sh = 1.62 Gz^{1/3} \quad (35)$$

$$Sh = 0.5 Gz \quad (36)$$

$$Gz = \mathrm{Re}\, Sc \frac{d_{in}}{L} \quad (37)$$

Where, d_{in} and L are internal diameter and fiber length, respectively. Likewise, a good correlation for shell side, considering the industrial modules configuration, is the Basu correlation (Basu et al., 1990; Yun et al., 1993),

$$Sh = 17.4(1-\phi)\frac{d_h}{L}\mathrm{Re}^{0.6}\, Sc^{0.33} \quad (38)$$

$$\phi = n\left[\frac{d_{out}}{D_{in}}\right]^2 \tag{39}$$

In the above equations, d_h is the hydraulic diameter (4 x flow area/wet perimeter), the solution flow velocity in the shell side is determined by flow area/hydraulic diameter, d_{out} is the external diameter of the fibers, D_{in} is the internal diameter of the shell and n is the number of the fibers in the membrane module.

On the other hand, the local mass transfer coefficient for the membrane pore can be assumed as a molecular diffusion process (Gabelman and Hwang, 1999) as shown in Equation 40.

$$k = \frac{D_{HCN-P}\varepsilon}{\tau e} \tag{40}$$

Where $D_{HCN\text{-}P}$ is the diffusion coefficient of HCN in the phase which fills the pore, ε is porosity, τ is tortuosity, and e is fiber thickness. A summary of different correlations for common systems that generate gaseous HCN is presented in Table 4.

The estimation of the local mass transfer coefficients requires the determination of the physical properties of the liquid and gas phases, such as density and viscosity. Due to the low HCN concentrations in the liquid and gas phase, both physical properties are assumed similar to those specified for water and air, respectively. These physical properties are estimated by using empirical and semi-empirical models controlled by the operational conditions of the system. Thus, for the air phase, the density can be calculated by the ideal gas law (Smith et al., 2005), while the viscosity can be estimated by the Chapman-Enskog's model (Bird et al., 2007) or by using empirical data (Perry and Green, 1997). Likewise, experimental data of density and viscosity for the liquid phase obtained from Perry and Green (1997) has been correlated as a function of temperature by Estay et al. (2007).

Table 4. Local mass transfer correlations for different systems.

Physical system	Correlation	Parameters	Range	Flow pattern	Equation	Source
Flat plate	$Sh = 0.664\ \mathrm{Re}^{0.5}\ Sc^{1/3}$	L_C=Plate length	Re<50,000	Laminar flow condition	29	Treybal, 1980
	$Sh = 0.023\mathrm{Re}^{0.83}\ Sc^{1/3}$		Re>50,000	Turbulent flow condition	30	Treybal, 1980
Agitated tanks	$Sh = 0.13\left[\frac{L_C^4 (W/V)\rho^2}{\mu^3}\right]^{1/4} Sc^{1/3}$	L_C=Tank length W/V=Power per tank volume ratio	-	-	31	Cussler, 2009
Natural convection	$k_P = \frac{D_{HCN-P}}{z}$	z=Boundary layer	-	Natural convection	32	Treybal, 1980
Packed beds	$\frac{k_P}{v^0} = 1.17\left(\frac{d_p v^0 \rho}{\mu}\right)^{-0.42}\left(\frac{\mu}{\rho D_{HCN^{-}-P}}\right)^{-0.67}$	v^0=superficial velocity $d_p = \frac{6(1-\varepsilon)}{a}$	-	-	33	Cussler, 2009
Lumen side of membranes contactors	$Sh = 1.62 Gz^{1/3}$ $Sh = 0.5 Gz$	$Gz = \mathrm{Re}\ Sc \frac{d_{in}}{L}$ d_{in}=Internal diameter of fibers L=Fiber length	Gz>6 Gz<6	Laminar flow conditions	35 36	Shen et al., 2010
Shell side of membranes contactors	$Sh = 17.4(1-\phi)\frac{d_h}{L}\mathrm{Re}^{0.6}\ Sc^{0.33}$	$\phi = n\left[\frac{d_{out}}{D_{in}}\right]^2$ d_h=Hydraulic diameter d_{out}=External diameter of fibers D_{in}=Shell diameter	-	Laminar flow conditions	38	Basu et al., 1990

Table 4. (continued).

Physical system	Correlation	*Parameters*	Range	Flow pattern	Equation	Source
Membrane pores	$k = \frac{D_{HCN-P}\varepsilon}{\tau e}$	ε=Porosity τ=Tortuosity e=Fiber thickness	-	-	40	Gabelman and Hwang, 1999
Flow through circular pipe	$Sh = 1.62Gz^{1/3}$ $Sh = 0.023\mathrm{Re}^{0.83}Sc^{1/3}$	L_C=Pipe diameter	Re<2,100 Re>4,000	Laminar flow condition Turbulent flow condition	41 42	Bird et al., 2007 Treybal, 1980
Flow around a sphere	$Sh = 2.0 + 0.6\mathrm{Re}^{0.5}Sc^{1/3}$ $Sh = 2.0 + 0.6Gr^{0.25}Sc^{1/3}$	$Gr = \frac{d^3\rho\Delta\rho g}{\mu^2}$	-	Forced convection Natural convection	43 44	Cussler, 2009

3.3. Diffusion Coefficients of Hydrogen Cyanide

The most significant physical parameter in the hydrogen cyanide transfer is the diffusion coefficient in both phases involved in the process (gas and liquid). In this context, it seems strange the limited experimental data reported in literature for the diffusion coefficient of HCN in air and water. Klotz and Miller (1947) determined found a diffusion coefficient ($D_{HCN\text{-}air}$) of 0.173 cm^2/s at 0ºC and 1 atm, and Lotter (2006) adapted the HCN diffusion coefficient in water ($D_{HCN\text{-}water}$) from Dodge and Zabban (1952), obtaining a value of 1.72 x 10^{-5} cm^2/s at 20ºC. These values (summarized in Table 5) have been reported by other sources, but there is no additional information about experimental data for different conditions of pressure and temperature.

Table 5. Experimental data of diffusion coefficients for HCN in water and air.

Diffusion coefficient	Units	Conditions	Value	Source
$D_{HCN\text{-}water}$	cm^2/s	20°C	1.72 x 10^{-5}	Lotter, 2006
$D_{HCN\text{-}air}$	cm^2/s	0°C 1 atm	0.173	Klotz and Miller, 1947

The limited data reported for diffusion coefficient of HCN has forced the use of the semi-empirical equations reported in literature (Cussler, 2009; Bird et al., 2007; Poling et al., 2001) in order to estimate diffusion coefficients. The most common model for the estimation of gaseous diffusion coefficient was developed by Chapman & Enskog (Cussler, 2009):

$$D_{AB} = \frac{1.86 \cdot 10^{-3} T^{3/2} (1/M_A + 1/M_B)^{1/2}}{P \sigma_{AB}^2 \Omega} \tag{45}$$

Here, D_{AB} is the diffusion coefficient (cm^2/s), M_A and M_B are the molecular weights for compound A and B, respectively, P is the system pressure (atm), T is absolute temperature (K), and Ω and σ_{AB} are the Lennard-Jones molecular properties. The collision diameter σ_{AB}, in angstroms, is represented by:

$$\sigma_{AB} = \frac{1}{2}(\sigma_A + \sigma_B) \tag{46}$$

Values of collision diameter for air and hydrogen cyanide are 3.711 and 3.63 angstroms, respectively (Poling et al., 2001). Also, Ω is the diffusion collision integral, given by the following expression reported by Poling et al. (2001).

$$\Omega = \frac{1.06036}{(kT/\varepsilon_{AB})^{0.1561}} + \frac{0.193}{\exp(0.47635kT/\varepsilon_{AB})} + \frac{1.03587}{\exp(1.52996kT/\varepsilon_{AB})} + \frac{1.76474}{\exp(3.89411kT/\varepsilon_{AB})} \quad (47)$$

The energy parameter ε_{AB} is a geometric average of contributions of the two species:

$$\varepsilon_{AB} = (\varepsilon_A + \varepsilon_B)^{1/2} \quad (48)$$

The values of ε_i/k for air and HCN are 78.6 and 569.1 K, respectively (Poling et al., 2001). Thus, the result of estimating the diffusion coefficient of HCN in air with these equations, for 0°C and 1 atm, is 0.13 cm^2/s, obtaining 25% error. There are other equations for calculation of the gaseous diffusion value, such as Fuller model and Wilkee and Lee model (Cussler, 2009; Poling et al., 2001), probably with higher accurate than the Chapman Enskog model, although the effect of temperature and pressure in the diffusion coefficient values at low pressures are identical in these models. Therefore, it is possible to specify the $D_{HCN\text{-}air}$ for other temperature and pressure conditions using the experimental value reported:

$$\frac{D_{HCN-air}(T_1, P_1)}{D_{HCN-air}(T_1, P_2)} = \frac{T_1^{3/2} P_2}{T_2^{3/2} P_1} \quad (49)$$

Otherwise, the diffusion coefficient for HCN in water can be estimated by semi-empirical equations, such as Sutherland equation, Glasstone equation, Scheibel equation, Wilke and Chang equation, Tyn and Calus equation, Hayduk, and Minhas correlation (Cussler, 2009; Poling et al., 2001). These equations are based on the Stokes-Einstein equation shown in the following expression:

$$D_{AB} = \frac{k_B}{6\pi\mu R_0} \quad (50)$$

Where, k_B is the Boltzmann's constant, R_0 is the radius of the "spherical" solute and μ is the viscosity of the solvent. The Wilke-Chang equation is one of the most used equations to estimate diffusion coefficients in liquids. Equation (51) shows this model.

$$D_{AB} = \frac{7.4 \cdot 10^{-8} (\Phi M_B)^{1/2} T}{\mu V_A^{0.6}} \tag{51}$$

Here, D_{AB} is the diffusion coefficient (cm^2/s), T is absolute temperature (K), M_B is the molecular weight of the solvent (g/mol), μ is the viscosity of the solvent (cP), Φ is the association factor of the solvent B (dimensionless) - 2.6 for water- , and V_A is the molar volume of the solute at its normal boiling temperature (cm^3/mol). Using this equation to estimate the diffusion coefficient of HCN in water at 20°C results a value of 1.26 x 10^{-5} cm^2/s, obtaining 26% error in the estimation. Hence, similarly to HCN diffusion in air, the HCN diffusion coefficient in water can be determined from experimental data dependent on water temperature and viscosity. Considering the above value, the HCN diffusion coefficient in water for different conditions can be determined by:

$$\frac{D_{HCN-liq}(T_1)}{D_{HCN-liq}(T_2)} = \frac{T_1 \mu_2}{T_2 \mu_1} \tag{52}$$

Independently of the accuracy of the used method for calculation of the diffusion coefficient, it is important to make mention of the fact that the difference of values between the diffusion coefficient of HCN in air and in water is approximately four orders of magnitude. Therefore, the mass transfer of HCN in the liquid phase will be the controlling step of HCN gas generation in any process.

4. Hydrogen Cyanide Gas Generation in Different Systems

The model proposed in this work for gaseous HCN generation is based on the theoretical background described above, and the design parameters for the equipment units involved in this kind of operations. All equations were derived with the aim of determining the HCN transferred from cyanide solution into the air and the HCN concentration reached in the air. The model constructed could be applied to the main equipment or systems currently operating in cyanidation processes.

4.1. Assumptions

In order to apply the simulation model proposed here, some specific considerations and assumptions were introduced into the theoretical approach:

a) The process is considered isothermal, operating under steady-state conditions or batch conditions. When a batch process is used, the time variable must be employed.
b) This model is only useful for diluted systems, considering that the the most common situations for cyanide-using systems are diluted aqueous solutions and air.
c) Physical properties of water were used to define the physical properties of the liquid phase.
d) The physical properties of air were used to define the physical properties of the gas phase.

4.2. Numerical Solution of the Model

The model of HCN gas generation was evaluated by a numerical algorithm that estimates the transferred HCN from cyanide solution into the air for any equipment. This algorithm estimates the HCN transfer by comparing the value obtained from the resistances-in-series mass transfer model and the cyanide mass balance described by Equations (53-54). When the difference between the HCN transferred values is lower than the set target, the iterative routine is finished.

$$N_{HCN} = FC_{HCNL\,inlet} - FC_{HCNL\,outlet} \tag{53}$$

$$-\frac{d(VC_{HCNL\,t})}{dt} = F(C_{HCNL\,t} - C_{HCNL\,inlet}) + N_{HCN} \tag{54}$$

Here, F is the total solution flow, $C_{HCNLinlet}$ and $C_{HCNLoutlet}$ are the HCN concentrations in the inlet and outlet solution of equipment operating under steady-state condition, respectively, C_{HCNLt} is the HCN concentration in the solution at time t, and V is the volume accumulated in the inventory stock.

Equation (53) represents a mass balance in steady state; therefore the algorithm compares the solution of mass transfer model and Equation (53). Besides, Equation (54) represents the mass balance in dynamic systems, where inventory of cyanide in a system is observed. The algorithm solves dynamic conditions by using Equation (54) for each time, estimating profiles of HCN mass transfer rate (N_{HCN}) and concentration as function of time. Another solution method for the dynamic problem is integrating Equation (54) to obtain an equation of HCN concentration as function of time. A mass balance for gas phase can be similarly developed to Equations (53-54).

The steady-state condition is the most common situation in the industry, but a dynamic estimation is useful to obtain profiles of HCN transferred in tailings dams, cyanide ponds in heap leaching processes, accumulation tanks, among others. In this context, the simplest system to solve the dynamic problem is found in static tanks or dams, where it can be supposed constant HCN content in the liquid phase for a determined time, and HCN concentration in the gas phase around 0 ppm. Equation (55) shows the solution of Equation (54) for this simple system.

$$\ln\left(\frac{C_{HCNL\,t}}{C_{HCN\,0}}\right) = -\frac{K_L A t}{V} \tag{55}$$

Here, the evolution of HCN concentration in the liquid phase, as function of time (C_{HCNt}) is dependent of the initial HCN concentration (C_{HCN0}), containment volume (V), global mass transfer coefficient (K_L), and mass transfer area (A).

The results of the model can be reported as evaporated HCN mass in equipment and HCN concentration in the gas phase. Finally, the numerical algorithm was developed in Matlab® language using similar considerations from previous works (Estay et al., 2007; Estay et al., 2012). If the Matlab® language is not available for users, other computational tools (for example, Excel) can be used.

In order to highlight potential applications of the model proposed in this work, the following sections illustrate the estimation of gaseous HCN generated in different systems: tank without agitation in steady state, tank without agitation with air stream flowing on the top in steady state, and agitated tank with air stream flowing on the top in steady state.

4.3. HCN Gas Generation in a Tank without Agitation in Steady State

Cyanidation processes include many tanks without agitation, such as pumping tanks, feed tanks, and transfer tanks, which could generate HCN according to the operational conditions. Figure 6 shows an schematic diagram of a tank without agitation fed with a solution containing 600 mg/L total cyanide, 250 mg/L copper, and 80 mg/L nickel at 15°C, solution with the same composition that that one characterized in Figure 2. The design parameters of the tank are shown in Table 6. Additionally, the mass transfer correlations used for this case correspond to natural convection (Equation 32) for both phases, since the systems are operated without agitation. Thus, the results of HCN gas generation in this system are presented as HCNconcentration in the air and the HCN transferred ratio (mass of HCN transferred from solution into the air per mass transfer area, mg/h m^2). The impact of pH on the HCN gas generation is shown in Figure 7.

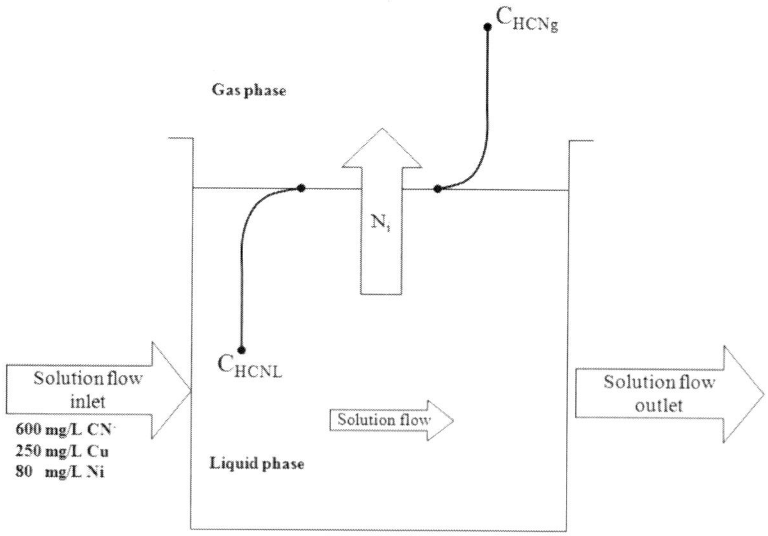

Figure 6. Schematic diagram of the tank without agitation, considering natural convection in both phases (liquid and gas).

Table 6. Design parameters and operational conditions of the system evaluated.

Parameter	Value	Unit
T	15	°C
P	550	mmHg
$[CN]_T$	600	mg/L
[Cu]	250	mg/L
[Ni]	80	mg/L
V	60	m^3
Diameter-Length ratio	1	-
F	200	m^3/h

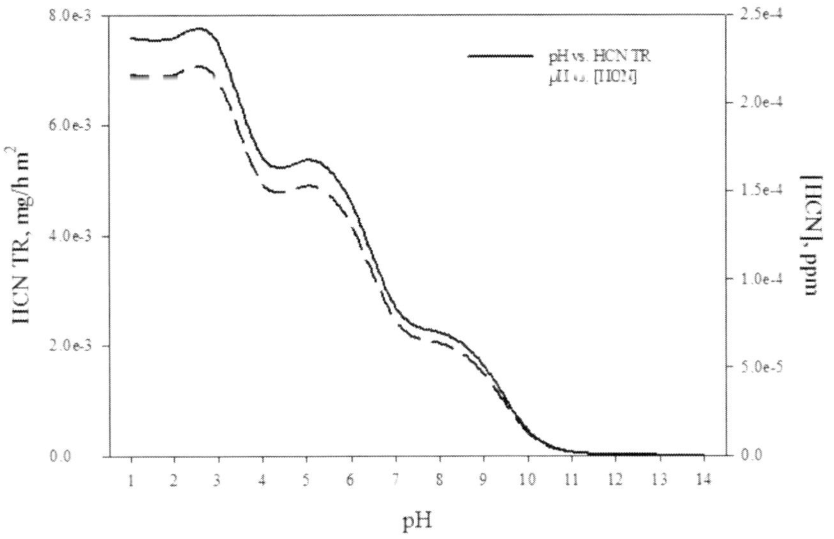

Figure 7. HCN transferred ratio (HCN TR) and HCN concentration in the gas phase as function of pH in the tank without agitation, considering natural convection in both phases.

The HCN concentration in the air and the HCN transferred ratio are decreased when pH increases due to the effect of pH in the dissociation of metals-cyanide species, determining the HCN concentration in the solution (see Figure 2) and consequently limiting the HCN transfer into the air. Thus, the HCN transferred ratio decreases from 0.0080 to 0.0005 mg/(h m^2) when pH increases from 3 to 10, and the HCN concentration obtained in the air is lower than 2.2 x 10^{-4} ppm, value under the limit established by local regulations (around 4.7 ppm). These low values of HCN concentration in the air and HCN transferred ratio are explained by the high mass transfer resistance of the process, promoted by the low local mass transfer coefficients obtained in the process (7.5×10^{-9} m/s for liquid phase, and 1.3×10^{-4} m/s for gas phase), which depend on the system turbulence, almost negligible in this process.

4.4. HCN Gas Generation in a Tank without Agitation with Air Stream Flowing on the Top in Steady State

Another system that could be found in cyanidation processes is similar to the above mentioned, considering a sealed tank with an air stream flowing onto the liquid-gas interface, in order to drag the HCN contained in the air. Figure 8 shows a schematic diagram of a sealed tank without agitation with air stream flowing on the top, receiving the same solution that the previous case. This tank is identical to the one described in section 4.3, considering a free space between the liquid-gas interface and the seal of the tank, 0.25 m. On the other hand, the mass transfer correlations for this case apply for natural convection (Equation 32) in the liquid phase and flat plate (Equations 29 and 30) for the gas phase, considering air flowing parallel to the liquid-gas interface and a flat surface. Therefore, in order to evaluate the impact of air flow in the HCN transfer, the results of the HCN gas concentration in the air and HCN transferred ratio are presented in Figure 9, as function of air flow-liquid flow volumetric ratio.

The HCN gas generation increased less than 1% when the air flow-liquid flow volumetric ratio increased from 0.5 to 5.0, according to Figure 9. Also, the values of the HCN transferred ratio were around 0.0054 mg/(h m^2). According to the above results, the air flow-liquid flow volumetric ratio induces a minor impact on the HCN gas generation. This behaviour is determined by the distribution of the local mass transfer resistances, which were estimated as a quotient between the value of the local mass transfer coefficient and the overall mass transfer coefficient. This system presented local mass transfer resistances in the liquid phase higher than 99.99%.

Besides, the air flow determines the HCN concentration in the gas phase. As expected, the HCN concentration decreased when the air flow-liquid flow volumetric ratio was increased. This outcome is determined by the dilution effect induced by the air flow. Moreover, the HCN concentration in the tank was lower than 9×10^{-4} ppm. Thus, values of HCN concentration below 4.7

ppm are not considered dangerous for personnel in case of air leaks or direct exposure.

The HCN transferred ratio in this system is slightly higher than the system evaluated earlier, because of the highest values of the gas phase coefficient.

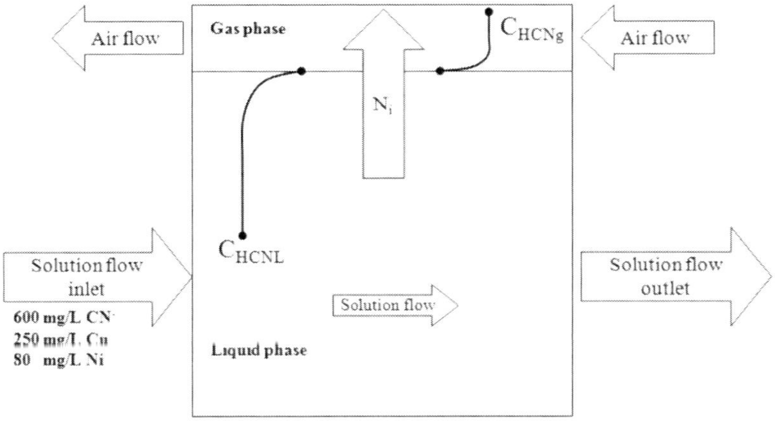

Figure 8. Schematic diagram of the tank without agitation, considering natural convection in liquid phase and forced convection in the gas phase.

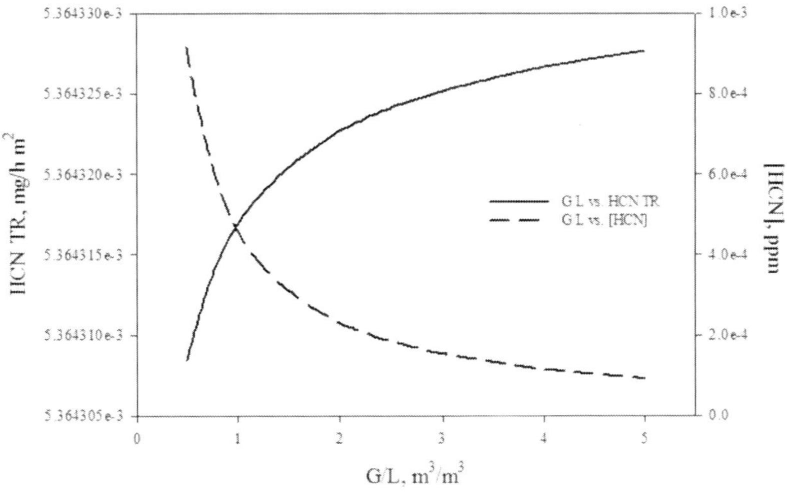

Figure 9. HCN transferred ratio (HCN TR) and HCN concentration in the gas phase at pH 5 as function of air flow-liquid flow volumetric ratio in the tank without agitation, considering natural convection in liquid phase and forced convection in gas phase.

4.5. HCN Gas Generation in an Agitated Tank with Air Stream Flowing on the Top in Steady State

Reactors and agitated tanks are common equipment units in cyanidation processes and cyanide recovery processes. These systems comprise a mechanic agitator in the liquid phase, and natural or forced convection in the gas phase. For purposes of this analysis, the tank simulated is mechanically agitated in the liquid phase, sealed with air stream flowing onto the liquid phase. Figure 10 shows a schematic diagram of this system (similar tosection 4.4), receiving the same solution of the previous cases. Additionally, the mass transfer correlations used for this case are the agitated tank correlations (Equation 31) for liquid phase and flat plate (Equations 29 and 30) for the gas phase, considering air flowing in counter-current over the liquid-gas interface. In order to evaluate the effect of the turbulence on the liquid phase, the results of HCN gas concentration in the air and HCN transferred ratio are presented in Figure 11 as function of power/tank volume ratio.

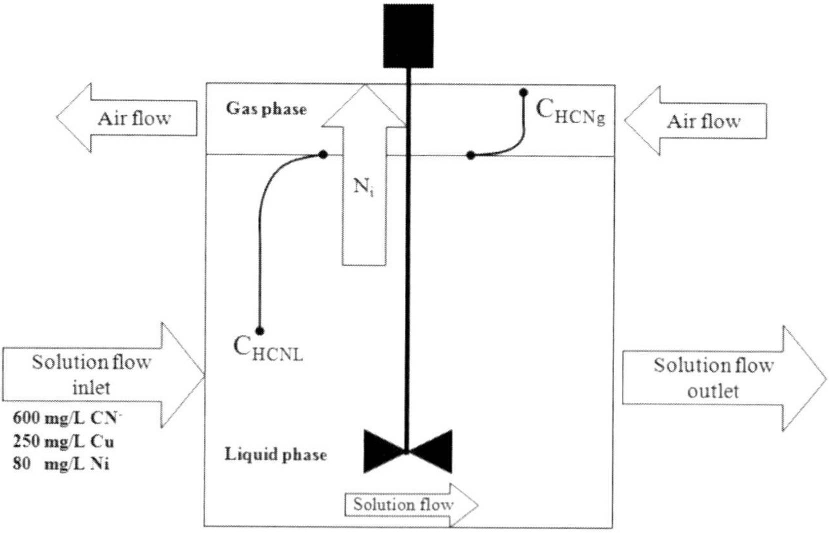

Figure 10. Schematic diagram of the agitated tank, considering forced convection both phases.

Figure 11 shows that an increase in the agitation power-tank volume ratio from 50 to 500 W/m^3 produces an increase in the HCN transferred ratio around 77%, due to the increase of the local mass transfer coefficient in the liquid phase, reducing the liquid mass transfer resistance. Therefore, the power agitation/tank volume ratio is a relevant design parameter involved in the HCN gas generation. On the other hand, the HCN concentration in this system is lower than 1 ppm, for an air flow-liquid flow volumetric ratio value of 3.0 m^3/m^3.

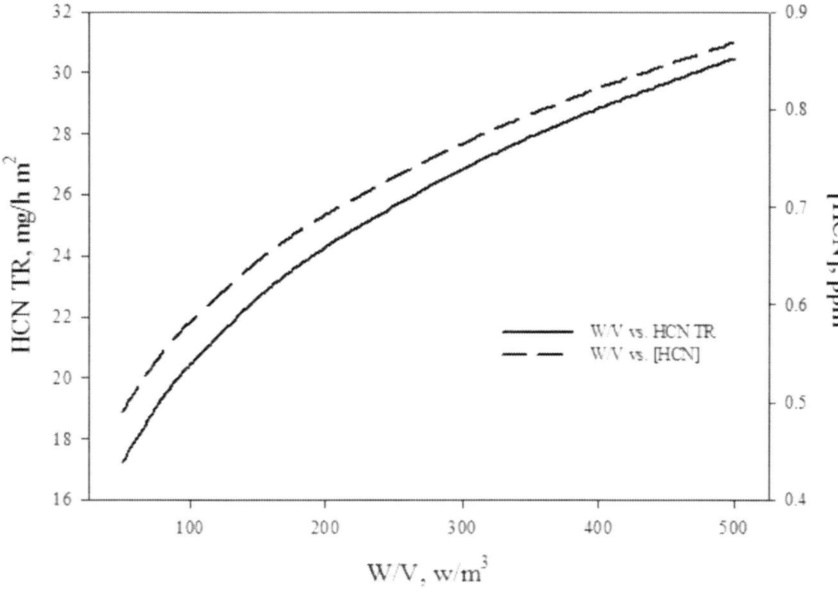

Figure 11. HCN transferred ratio (HCN TR) and HCN concentration in the gas phase as function of power-tank volume ratio in the agitated tank, considering forced convection in both phases, air flow-liquid flow volumetric ratio of 3.0 m^3/m^3, at pH 5.

Hence, the HCN concentration values for the evaluated systems do not represent risk for personnel, according to the current regulations; however, to reduce and control the HCN emanations, design parameters and operational conditions must be adequately addressed.

4.6. The Effect of Total Cyanide Concentration on the HCN Gas Generation

The total cyanide concentration determines the HCN gas generation in a process, according to the mass transfer model (Equations 21 and 21a). Figure 12 shows the effect of the total cyanide concentration on the HCN transferred ratio and HCN concentration in the gas phase for the agitated tank presented in the earlier section (Figure 10), keeping the copper and nickel concentrations constant. The behaviour presented in Figure 12 shows an increase of HCN transferred ratio from 9.0 to 271 mg/(hm^2) when the total cyanide concentration is increased from 400 to 5,000 mg/L, and the HCN concentration is higher than the limit established (4.7 ppm) for total cyanide concentrations greater than 3,200 mg/L. These values are explained by the increase of the HCN content in the solution and the proportionality of the HCN concentration gradient in the mass transfer rate (Equations 21 and 21a).

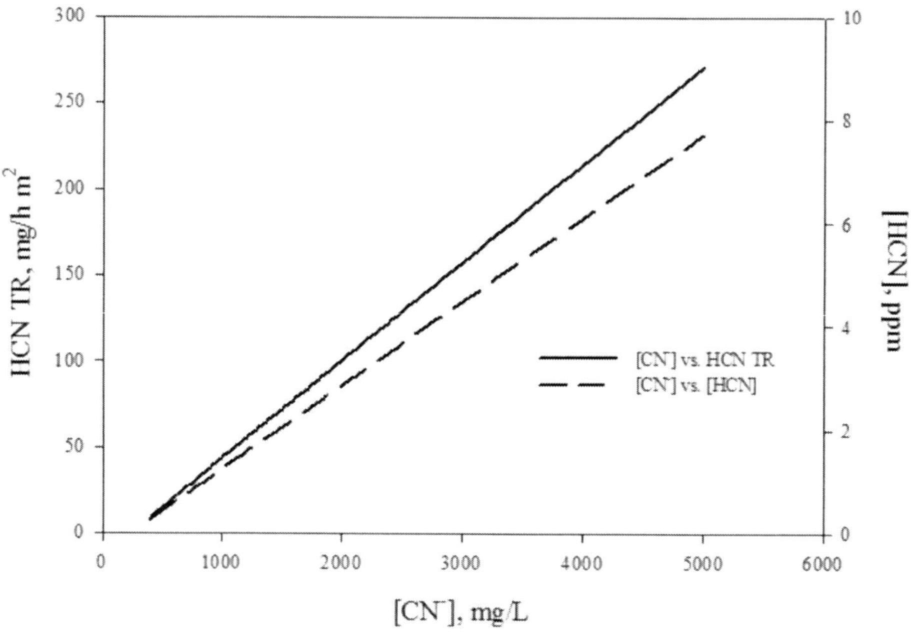

Figure 12. HCN transferred ratio (HCN TR) and HCN concentration in the gas phase as function of total cyanide concentration in the feed solution ([CN^-]) in the agitated tank, considering forced convection in both phases, at pH 5 air flow-liquid flow volumetric ratio equal to 3.0 m^3/m^3 and a power agitation-tank volume ratio of 100 W/m^3.

The overall results presented here lead to the conclusion that specific simulation models for each system or operational condition are needed to evaluate cyanide contents that could induce risks to workers, predicting dangerous conditions and evaluating possible actions for taking the process forward.

5. Future Trends

The current regulations for HCN contents in the workplaces, leach tails, tailings dams, wastewaters, among others, have forced to the industries that use or produce cyanide to increase the safety standards in their processes, including new unit operations, andeliminate cyanide contents in the wastewaters or tailings. Hereafter, the plant design and the operational control of these processes must include parameters or measurements that avoidrisk of hydrogen cyanide emanations. In this context, the present work can be used in the early stages of the process design to identify risk conditions in a unit operation, and proposing the modifications that minimize risk conditions. Additionally, the current operations can use this model to identify and put attention on the risk areas. Also, the thermodynamic characterization presented here is a powerful tool to understand the behaviour of cyanidation solutions in the processes, taking adequate decisions in order to optimize the operational conditions.

Conclusion

A general method has been presented here to predict the HCN gas generation in industrial processes as a function of operational parameters. According to the results obtained, the HCN gas generation is controlled by the liquid mass transfer resistance which presented values higher than 99% (of the total resistance) due to the four order of magnitude difference in the HCN diffusion coefficients between water and air (10-9 m^2/s vs. 10-5 m^2/s). This difference establishes that the liquid phase exerts a high mass transfer resistance, limiting the HCN transferred rate in the systems that have low agitation or turbulence. Additionally, the HCN concentrations in the air had values lower than 4.7 ppm (the limit established by regulations), for the systems and operational conditions studied, except for the total cyanide concentration higher than 3,200 mg/L, where the HCN transferred ratio increases over 170 mg/(h m^2). Hence, the adequate control of critical parameters could promote an increase of the local mass transfer in the liquid phase, being this point relevant to avoid the HCN gas generation.

Finally, this method can be applied to characterize any solution containing cyanide in a process. Therefore, the methodology presented here is useful for the characterization of metal-cyanide species in solution, predicting the HCN concentration in the air close to a unit operation, the losses of cyanide promoted by HCN degradation, and establishing the operational parameters most influential in a process.

References

Adams, M.D.; Fleming, C.A. *Metall Trans B.* 1989, 20B, 315-325.

Basu, R.; Prasad, R.; Sirkar, K.K. *AIChE J.* 1990, 36, 450-460.

Bird, R.; Stewart, W.; Lightfoot, E. *Transport Phenomena,* ISBN 0-470-11539-4; John Wiley and Sons: New York, NY, 2007.

Bodek, I.; Lyman, W.; Reehl, W.; Rosenblatt, D. *Environmental inorganic chemistry: properties, processes, and estimation methods,* ISBN 0-08-036833-6; Pergamon Press: New York, NY, 1988.

Christensen, J.; Izzat, R.; Eatough, D. *Inorg Chem.* 1965, 4, 1278-1280.

Christensen, J.; Izzat, R.; Hale, *J. Inorg Chem.* 1963, 2, 337-339.

Cussler, E. *Diffusion: Mass Transfer in Fluid Systems,* ISBN 978-0-521-87121-1; Cambridge University Press: Cambridge, UK, 2009.

Dodge, B.; Zabban, W. *Plat Surf Finish.* 1952, 29, 1133-1139.

Dzombak, D.A.; Ghosh, R.S.; Young, T.S. In *Cyanide in Water and Soil: Chemistry, Risk and Management*; Dzombak, D.A.; Ghosh, R.S.; Wong-Chong, G.M.; ISBN-10 1-56670-666-1; CRC Taylor and Francis Group: Boca Raton, FL, 2006, pp 57-92.

Estay, H.; Ortiz, M.; Romero, J. A process based on gas filled membrane absorption to recover cyanide in gold mining. Accepted by *Hydrometallurgy.* 2013.

Estay, H.; Becker, J.; Carvajal, P.; Arriagada, F. *Hydrometallurgy.* 2012, 113-114, 131-142.

Estay, H.; Hasanoğlu, A.; Romero, J. Gas-filled membrane absorption: A novel process to recover cyanide in gold cyanidation. In *XXV Interamerican Congress of Chemical Engineering (CIIQ 2011),* Santiago, Chile, 2011.

Estay, H.; Bocquet, S.; Romero, J.; Sanchez, J.; Rios, G.M.; Valenzuela, F. *Chem Eng Sci.* 2007, 62, 5794-5808.

Fleming, C.A. *Dev Miner Process.* 2005, 15, 703-727.

Gabelman, A.; Hwang, S-T. *J Membr Sci.* 1999, 159, 61-106.

Geankopolis, C. *Transport Processes and Unit Operations,* ISBN 0139304398; Prentice Hall PTR: New Jersey, NJ, 1993.

Ghosh, R.S.; Dzombak, D.A.; Wong-Chong, G.M.. In *Cyanide in Water and Soil: Chemistry, Risk and Management;* Dzombak, D.A.; Ghosh, R.S.; Wong-Chong, G.M.; ISBN-10 1-56670-666-1; CRC Taylor and Francis Group: Boca Raton, FL, 2006, pp 15-23.

Izzat, R.; Dee Johnston, H.; Watt, G.; Christensen, *J. Inorg Chem.* 1967, 6, 132-135.

Izzat, R.; Christensen, J.; Hansen, J.; Watt, G. *Inorg Chem.* 1965, 4, 718-721.

Izzat, R.; Christensen, J.; Pack, R.; Bench, R. *Inorg Chem.* 1962, 1, 828-831.

Klotz, I.; Miller, D. *J Am Chem Soc.* 1947, 69(10), 2557-2558

Logsdon, M.; Hagelstein, K.; Mudder, T. *The Management of Cyanide in Gold Extraction*, ISBN 1-895720-27-3; International Council on Metals and the Environment: Ontario, 1999.

Lotter, N. *Cyanide volatilization from gold leaching operations and tailing storage facilities.* Thesis to obtain a master's degree in Metallurgical Engineering, Faculty of Engineering, Built Environment and Information Technology, University of Pretoria, Republic of South Africa. 2006.

Lu, J.; Dreisinger, D.; Cooper, W. *Hydrometallurgy.* 2002, 66, 23-36.

Ma, J.; Dasgupta, P.; Blackledge, W.; Boss, G. *Environ Sci Technol*, 2010, 44, 3028-3034.

McCabe, W.; Smith, J.; Harriott, P. *Unit Operations of Chemical Engineering*, ISBN 0-07-284823-5; McGraw-Hill: New York, NY, 2004.

Marsden, J.O.; House, C.I. The Chemistry of Gold Extraction, ISBN-10 0-87335-240-8; *Society for Mining, Metallurgy and Exploration SME*: Littleton, CO, 2006.

Mudder, T.I.; Botz, M.M. *Eur J Miner Process Environ Prot.* 2004, 4, 62-74.

Perry, R.; Green, D.; Maloney, J. *Perry's Chemical Engineers' Handbook*, ISBN 0-07-049841-5; McGraw-Hill: New York, NY, 1997.

Poling, B.; Prausnitz, J.; O'Connell, J. *The Properties of Gases and Liquids*, ISBN 0-07-011682-2; McGraw-Hill: New York, NY, 2001.

Senanayake, G. *Hydrometallurgy.* 2008, 90, 46-73.

Shen, S.; Kentish S.; Stevens, G. *Solvent Extr Ion Exc.* 2010, 28, 817-844.

Smith, A.; Mudder, T. *The Chemistry and Treatment of Cyanidation Wastes,* ISBN 0-90-011751-6; Mining Journal Books Limited: London, 1991.

Smith, J.; Van Ness, H.; Abbott, M. *Introduction to Chemical Engineering Thermodynamics*, ISBN 0-07-310445-0; McGraw-Hill: New York, NY, 2005.

Treybal, R. *Mass Transfer Operations*, ISBN 0-07-065176-0; McGraw-Hill, New York, NY, 1980.

Watt, G.; Christensen, J.; Izzat, R. *Inorg Chem.* 1965, 4, 220-222.

Xue, T.; Osseo-Asare, K. *Metall Trans B*. 1985, 16B, 455-463.

Young, T.S.; Zhao, X.; Theis, T.L. *In Cyanide in Water and Soil: Chemistry, Risk and Management;* Dzombak, D.A.; Ghosh, R.S.; Wong-Chong, G.M.; ISBN-10 1-56670-666-1; CRC Taylor and Francis Group: Boca Raton, FL, 2006, pp 171-190.

Yun, C.H.; Prasad, R.; Guha, A.K.; Sirkar, K.K. *Ind. Eng. Chem. Res*. 1993, 32, 1186-1195.

In: Cyanide
Editor: Benito Soto-Blanco
ISBN: 978-1-62618-297-4

Chapter 4

APPLICATION OF CYANIDE-BRIDGED COORDINATION POLYMERS FOR ELECTRODE MATERIALS OF RECHARGEABLE BATTERIES

Masashi Okubo
National Institute of Advanced Industrial Science and Technology, Japan

ABSTRACT

Development of novel host materials with enhanced ion storage ability is of particular importance in a wide range of applications, especially the electrode materials for batteries. A cyanide-bridged coordination polymer is one of the most attractive host materials, because both the ionic-diffusion channel and electron conduction path frequently coexist within the framework. For example, a cyanide-bridged perovskite-type framework, so-called Prussian blue analog (PBA), has been studied intensively for decades from the viewpoint of electrochromism. However, the electrochemical properties, *i.e.*, electrochemical ion intercalation/extraction of PBAs can also be applied to the electrode materials of the batteries. In this chapter, the solid state electrochemistry of PBA is briefly explained. Then, the cyanide-bridged coordination polymer electrodes for the battery application are reviewed.

1. PRUSSIAN BLUE ANALOGS

In 1704, a new blue pigment for paints and fabrics was discovered. This pigment is now called Prussian blue (PB) or Berlin blue, which is the first synthetic coordination compound. PB and its analogs (PBAs) have the perovskite related structure, in which the octahedral metal centers are bridged by cyanide [1]. The formula is $A_xM[M'(CN)_6]_{1-y}\cdot\square_y\cdot nH_2O$ (A: alkali meta cation, M, M': transition metal, hereafter denoted as MM'-PBA, □: $[M'(CN)_6]$ vacancy) [2,3]. In general, PBAs, synthesized by mixing M and $[M'(CN)_6]$ in aqueous solution, contain a large amount of the $[M'(CN)_6]$ vacancy (□) occupied with zeolitic water. For example, PB is synthesized by mixing Fe^{III} and $[Fe^{II}(CN)_6]^{4-}$ in aqueous solution, and has a formula of $K_{1-4y}Fe^{III}[Fe^{II}(CN)^6]_{1-y}\cdot\square_y\cdot nH_2O$. The amount of vacancy, y, depends largely on the synthetic condition.

It is well known that mixing Fe^{II} and $[Fe^{III}(CN)_6]^{3-}$ in aqueous solution gives the so-called 'soluble form' of PB or Turnbull's blue. However, because of rapid electron transfer from Fe^{II} to $[Fe^{III}(CN)_6]^{3-}$, 'soluble' PB and 'insoluble' PB are identical ($K_{1-4y}Fe^{III}[Fe^{II}(CN)^6]_{1-y}\cdot\square_y\cdot nH_2O$), which was confirmed by the Mössbauer spectroscopy [4]. There are many literatures describing that, based on the early interpretation, 'soluble' PB is $KFe^{III}[Fe^{II}(CN)_6]\cdot nH_2O$, and 'insoluble' PB is $Fe^{III}[Fe^{II}(CN)_6]_{3/4}\cdot nH_2O$. But it is clear that such a simple classification is not correct.

A limit composition (y = 0, PBAs without the vacancy) is obtained as the chemical compositions of $A_2M^{II}[M'^{II}(CN)_6]$, $AM^{II}[M'^{III}(CN)_6]$ and $M^{III}[M'^{III}(CN)_6]$ (Figure 1). Although the composition $AM^{II}[M'^{III}(CN)_6]$ (A: Rb^+, Cs^+) can be synthesized by adding aqueous solution of M^{II} to aqueous solution of $[M'^{III}(CN)_6]^{3-}$ and excess A^+, the composition $A_2M^{II}[M'^{II}(CN)_6]$ is rare, and has been obtained, for example, as $A_2Mn^{II}[Mn^{II}(CN)_6]$ (A: Na^+, K^+, Rb^+ and Cs^+) and $K_2Fe^{II}[Fe^{II}(CN)_6]$ [5,6]. The composition $M^{III}[M'^{III}(CN)_6]$ is also rare, and has been obtained as $Fe^{III}[Co^{III}(CN)_6]$ [7]. In PBAs without the vacancy, M is octahedrally coordinated by 6 N atoms while M' is octahedrally coordinated by 6 C atoms. The crystal structure of PBAs without the vacancy basically adopts the face-centered cubic (*fcc*) structure. $Cs_2Mn^{II}[Mn^{II}(CN)_6]$, $RbMn[Fe(CN)_6]$, and $Fe^{III}[Co^{III}(CN)_6]$ possess the *fcc* structure. However, the detailed crystallographic study on a series of $A_2Mn^{II}[Mn^{II}(CN)_6]$ revealed that the cubic structure distorts when the ionic radius of A^+ decreases from Cs^+ to Na^+ (Figure 1). $Rb_2Mn^{II}[Mn^{II}(CN)_6]$ and $K_2Mn^{II}[Mn^{II}(CN)_6]$ are monoclinic [5], while $Na_2Mn^{II}[Mn^{II}(CN)_6]$ is rhombohedral [6].

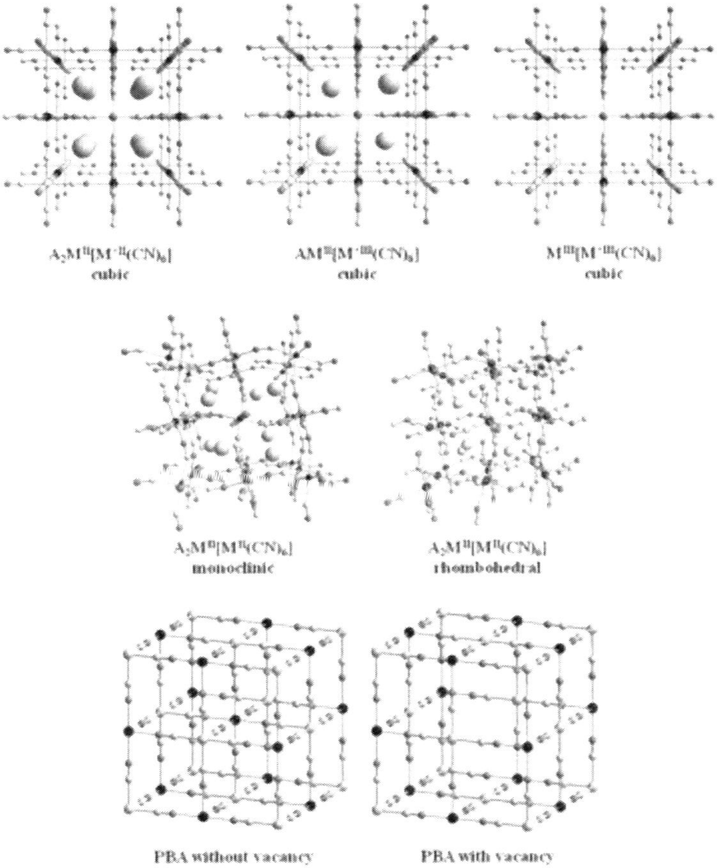

Figure 1. Crystal structure of various Prussian blue analogs $A_xM[M'(CN)_6]_{1-y}\cdot\square_y\cdot nH_2O$.

Nevertheless, the 3D framework, in which the octahedral metal centers are bridged by cyanide, is maintained in spite of the strong distortion from *fcc*.

PBAs with the vacancy ($y > 0$, $A_xM[M'(CN)_6]_{1-y}\cdot\square_y\cdot nH_2O$) is formed nominally by generating the Schottky-type defect of A^+ and $[M'(CN)_6]$ (Figure 1). The generated vacancy is occupied with the zeolitic water, and M is coordinated by N atoms of cyanide and O atoms of the coordinating water. For example, addition of 0.15 M Mn^{II} aqueous solution to 0.1 M $K_3[Fe^{III}(CN)_6]$ aqueous solution gives the composition $K_{0.1}Mn^{II}[Fe^{III}(CN)_6]_{0.7}\cdot\square_{0.3}\cdot 4.3H_2O$, in which 30% of the $[Fe^{III}(CN)_6]^{3-}$ site is vacant [8].

The electronic structure of PBAs is very intriguing, because of strong σ/π–donation and back donation between the transition metals and cyanide. The 3*d* orbital of the transition metals hybridizes well with 2*p* orbital of cyanide via metal-to-ligand or ligand-to-metal charge transferred states such as $d^{n-1}L$ or $d^{n+1}\underline{L}$ [9]. Here, L and $\underline{L}$ denote the ligand electron and hole, respectively. The hybridized molecular orbital allows the inter-valence charge transfer (IVCT), which is the origin of the bright blue color of PB [10]. By tuning the strong magnetic interaction between the metals through cyanide, magnetic properties of PBAs have been intensively investigated for decades. A room temperature ferrimagnet $V^{II}[Cr^{III}(CN)_6]_{0.86}\cdot\square_{0.14}\cdot 2.8H_2O$ was synthesized in 1995 [11]. In 1996, $K_{0.14}Co^{II/III}[Fe^{III/II}(CN)_6]_{0.71}\cdot\square_{0.29}\cdot 4.9H_2O$ was discovered to show an increase of both the magnetization and Curie temperature by light irradiation due to the IVCT, which is so-called photomagnetism [12]. The intriguing magnetic properties of PBAs were reviewed by M. Verdaguer [1,13] and S. Ohkoshi [14].

As shown in Figure 1, 3D porous open network exists in PBAs, in which A^+ can diffuse if the ionic radius of A^+ is smaller than the intercell bottleneck radius. Furthermore, an electron could move through the overlapping orbitals by thermally activated hopping as polaron. These two features provide PBAs with mixed conductivity to exhibit the topotactic electrochemical ion intercalation/extraction expressed as:

$$xA^+ + xe^- + PBA \leftrightarrow A_xPBA,$$

where A^+ is a cation such as Li^+, Na^+, K^+ and NH_4^+. Before discussing the application of the PBA electrodes, fundamentals of the solid state electrochemistry are explained briefly.

2. Solid State Electrochemistry of Prussian Blue Analogs

2.1. Solid State Electrochemistry

Solid state electrochemistry is not a new field of science, because it has an origin with the discovery of the first solid electrolyte PbF_2 and the first intercalation compound Ag_2S by M. Faraday [15]. Although liquid electrochemistry was developed dominantly, solid state electrochemistry has been attracting much attention since the 1960s, because both solid electrolytes and intercalation compounds are key technologies for the development of batteries and fuel cells. The Na^+ ion conductor sodium beta alumina was applied to the solid electrolyte in the Na/S batteries (1966, Ford Moter Company), while the proton conductor Nafion was used as the polymer electrolyte membrane in the polymer electrolyte fuel cell (PEFC) [16]. In 1976, M. S. Whittingham reported the Li^+ intercalation compound Li_xTiS_2, and proposed the concept of the rechargeable batteries based on the intercalation chemistry [17]. Soon afterward, Graphite/$LiCoO_2$ rocking chair battery, in which both anode and cathode materials are Li^+ intercalation compounds, was commercialized as a Li-ion battery in 1991 [18].

As mentioned in section 1, PBAs have the 3D-connected open porous cyanide-bridged framework, which is suitable for both the ionic diffusion and electronic conduction. The solid state electrochemistry, *i.e.*, electrochemical ion intercalation/extraction of PBAs was discovered by V. Neff in 1978 [19]. To date, the solid state electrochemistry of PBAs has been applied to various batteries as well as electrochromic devices. In this section, the thermodynamics of intercalation compounds is explained.

2.2. Thermodynamics of Intercalation Compounds

The number n_i of ion A in the host is one of the most important quantities in the thermodynamics of intercalation, because the Gibbs free energy G of the electrode material changes as a function of n_i. The chemical potential μ_i is defined as,

$$\mu_i = \frac{\partial G}{\partial n_i}\,. \tag{1}$$

Note that the chemical potential in the statistical mechanics is defined in the unit of eV per atom or molecule, while that in the thermodynamics is eV/mol. Since the ions in the host are treated by the statistical mechanics, the former is used in this chapter.

Consider an electrochemical cell with an intercalation electrode and a counter electrode. When the electric current passes through the cell with the potential difference E, the work done by the cell must equal to the change in the free energy of two electrodes as,

$$-zeE = \mu_i - \mu_C, \tag{2}$$

where z is the charge of ion, e is the elementary charge, and μ_C is the chemical potential of the counter electrode. If μ_C is kept constant (such as Li/Li^+ or Na/Na^+ or by using a reference electrode), E directly determines μ_i, which enables us to obtain μ_i as a function of the ion content x of A_x(host).

The chemical potential can be separated into a contribution from enthalpy H and entropy S as,

$$\mu_i = \frac{\partial H}{\partial n_i} - T\frac{\partial S}{\partial n_i} \tag{3}$$

Let us begin by assuming the intercalation electrode which shows the ion intercalation/extraction via a solid solution process in the composition range of $0 < x < 1$, and employ a lattice-gas model. In the lattice-gas model, each site of the lattice has two states as 'occupied' or 'vacant'. When ions are distributed over the sites, the configuration entropy of mixing is expressed by the Boltzmann equation,

$$S = k_B \ln W, \tag{4}$$

where k_B is the Boltzmann constant, and W is the number of states. When the ions are distributed randomly without interaction, W is,

$$W = \frac{N!}{n_i!(N-n_i)!}. \tag{5}$$

here, N is the number of the sites. By using the Stirling's approximation, the partial entropy as a function of x ($=\frac{n_i}{N}$) is,

$$\frac{\partial S}{\partial n_i} = -k_B \ln\frac{x}{1-x}. \tag{6}$$

Thus the chemical potential $\mu_i(x)$ is obtained as,

$$\mu_i = \frac{\partial H}{\partial n_i} + k_B T \ln\frac{x}{1-x}. \tag{7}$$

when the enthalpy term (the heat of mixing) is assumed as constant, the model describes the ions as ideal gas. However, when the ions are not ideal, theoretical expressions can most readily be obtained on the assumption that it is 'regular'. This model is so-called a regular solution model, in which the configuration entropy of mixing is still given by eq. (6), although the heat of mixing depends on x.

In the regular solution model, each site has a common neighboring number m. The number of the neighboring ion pair, which contributes to the enthalpy due to the interaction energy, is $\frac{1}{2}Nmx^2$. Thus, the chemical potential is modified by $\frac{\partial}{\partial n_i}(\frac{1}{2}JNmx^2)$ as,

$$\mu_i = \varepsilon + Jmx + k_B T \ln\frac{x}{1-x}, \tag{8}$$

where ε is x-independent site energy required for ion intercalation/extraction, and J is the interaction energy of the ion pair. This model is also called a mean field approximation, which is justified if $|J|$ is small enough. Therefore, the plot of $E(x)$ vs. x for the intercalation electrode is expressed as,

$$E(x) = E_0 - \frac{Jmx}{ze} - \frac{k_B T}{ze}\ln\frac{x}{1-x}. \tag{9}$$

The equation with $J = 0$ leads to the Nernst equation well known in the liquid electrochemistry. The higher order approximation for strong interaction has been developed by the Bethe approximation. The more complex host with non-equivalent sites has also been considered by the Lagrange multiplier.

In the regular solution model, $J > 0$ indicates repulsive interaction between ions while $J < 0$ indicates attractive interaction. The repulsive interaction between neighboring ions can be explained by the Coulombic interaction. On the other hand, an intercalated ion expands or contracts the lattice largely, giving rise to a strain field that decreases as the inverse square of the distance from the ion. The strain field results in an elastic interaction, which is frequently attractive to suppress the boundary formation.

Figure 2 shows the calculated $E(x)$ as a function of x based on eq. (9) with various J. The slope of the voltage decreases with increasing J. The simple mean-field expression helps us understand the intercalation compound just qualitatively, but there's a few examples such as $Li_xMo_6Se_8$ [20] or

$Li_x\{K_{0.2}Ni[Fe(CN)_6]_{0.7}\cdot\square_{0.3}\cdot4.7H_2O\}$ [21], in which the expression holds almost exactly.

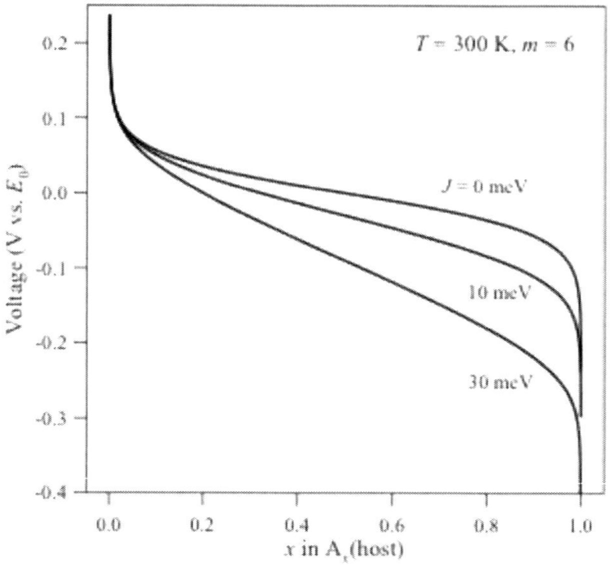

Figure 2. $E(x)$ vs. x for the host-guest system A_x(host) ($0 < x < 1$) according to eq. (9).

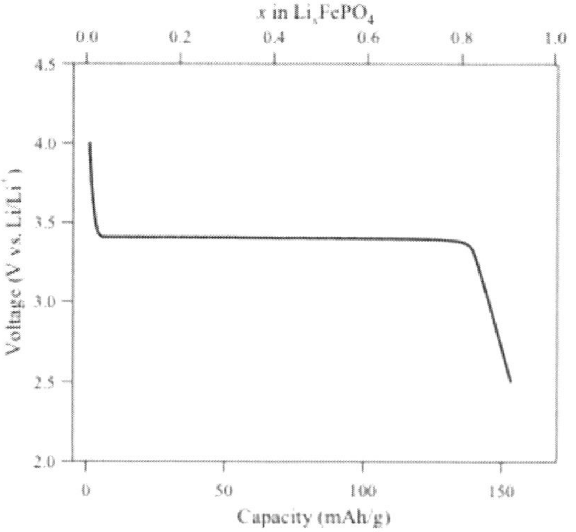

Figure 3. The voltage profile during Li^+ intercalation in Li_xFePO_4 through two-phase process.

Another important mechanism of ion intercalation/extraction is two phase process, where, during ion intercalation, domains of an ion rich phase grow at the expense of an ion poor phase. The two phase process frequently occurs when the elastic strain is too large to be accommodated with the host. A typical example is Li_xFePO_4[22], showing the two phase process as,

$$x\mathrm{Li}^+ + xe^- + \mathrm{FePO_4} \leftrightarrow (\mathrm{LiFePO_4})_x(\mathrm{FePO_4})_{1-x}.$$

here the solubility of Li^+ in each phase is ignored [23]. Li^+ intercalation results in the increase of the fraction of the Li rich $LiFePO_4$ phase. In the two phase systems, the enthalpy term in eq. (3) is constant while the entropy term is zero for the first approximation. Therefore, in contrast to the solid solution process, the voltage curve as a function of x is flat as shown in Figure 3. Nevertheless, the solid state electrochemistry of the two phase process should include various other factors such as coherency strain, anisotropic misfit strain, particle size (surface tension), temperature, and morphology. The interested readers can refer to the references [24-28].

In the liquid electrochemistry, the electrochemical reaction is usually studied by the current density as a function of E, for example, cyclic voltammetry (CV) or chronoamperometry, because the potential or kinetics of each electrochemical reaction is of main interest. In contrast, the solid state electrochemistry focuses on E as a function of the integrated specific current, which corresponds to x of A_x(host), because the thermodynamics of the electrode material is of primary interest. Therefore, although the CV is still important, most electrochemical experiments are performed galvanostatically, and E vs. x or E vs. specific capacity, so-called the charge-discharge curve, is usually employed to analyze the solid state electrochemical reaction.

The specific capacity in the unit of mAh/g (Ah/kg) is one of the most important intrinsic quantities of the intercalation compound, because it correlates with the specific energy of the battery (Wh/kg). Let us assume the electrochemical reaction, $xA^+ + xe^- + \text{host} \leftrightarrow A_x(\text{host})$, where the molar mass of the host is M [$g{\cdot}mol^{-1}$]. To fully reduce the host of 1g, the electric charge of $\frac{xF}{M}$ [C/g] should pass through the cell, where F is the Faraday constant. Since F is 96485 [C/mol], the theoretical capacity of the host is $\frac{26801x}{M}$ [mAh/g]. Therefore, in order to increase the specific energy of the batteries, the weight of the host per ion should be reduced.

2.3. Solid State Electrochemistry of PBAs

Early electrochemical works of PB were performed using K^+ aqueous electrolytes, and reported the electrochemical reaction with the nominal PB composition as:

$$K_2Fe^{II}[Fe^{II}(CN)_6] \leftrightarrow K^+ + e^- + KFe^{III}[Fe^{II}(CN)_6] \leftrightarrow 2K^+ + 2e^- + Fe^{III}[Fe^{III}(CN)_6],$$

because two pairs of reversible cathodic/anodic peaks were observed at 0.2 and 0.9 V vs. SCE in the CV [29,30]. According to these literatures, PB was reduced to Prussian white as the potential was made negative, while PB was oxidized to Prussian yellow or Berlin green as the potential was made positive. The above electrochemical reaction explained the CV of PB qualitatively: however, such a simple nominal composition is not correct, because PB and PBAs usually contain the vacancy as discussed in section 1. In the solid state electrochemistry, the composition of the electrode material is critical to determine the ion content x in the electrode, thus a precise composition of the electrode material must be used for the description of the solid state electrochemical reaction. The electrochemical reaction of PBAs is characterized into two extreme cases, *i.e.*, the redox of PBAs without the vacancy ($y = 0$) or redox of PBAs with the vacancy ($y > 0$). The former is expressed as,

$$\text{(i) } A^2M^{II}[M'^{II}(CN)_6] \leftrightarrow 2A^+ + 2e^- + M^{III}[M^{III}(CN)_6],$$

or

$$\text{(ii) } A'^+ + e^- + AM^{II}[M^{III}(CN)_6] \leftrightarrow A'AM^{II}[M'^{II}(CN)_6],$$

while the latter is expresses as,

$$\text{(iii) } (1\text{-}y)A'^+ + (1\text{-}y)e^- + A_xM[M'^{III}(CN)_6]_{1\text{-}y}\cdot\square_y\cdot nH_2O$$

$$\leftrightarrow A'_{1\text{-}y}A_xM[M'^{II}(CN)_6]_{1\text{-}y}\cdot\square_y\cdot nH_2O,$$

or

(iv) $A'^{+} + e^{-} + A_xM^{III}[M'^{II}(CN)_6]_{1-y}\cdot\square_y\cdot nH_2O \leftrightarrow A'A_xM^{II}[M'^{II}(CN)_6]_{1-y}\cdot\square_y\cdot nH_2O$.

Since PBAs without vacancy is rare, the latter two reactions have been mainly studied to date. The reaction types (ii), (iii) and (iv) correspond to the solid state redox of either C-coordinated or N-coordinated metal site, but further redox of another metal site is possible by extracting A^+. The electrochemical reaction of PB is classified into the reaction type (iv), but further redox of C-coordinated Fe occurs due to the accessible standard potential of $[Fe^{II}(CN)_6]^{4-}/[Fe^{III}(CN)_6]^{3-}$ redox couple, which well explains the CV.

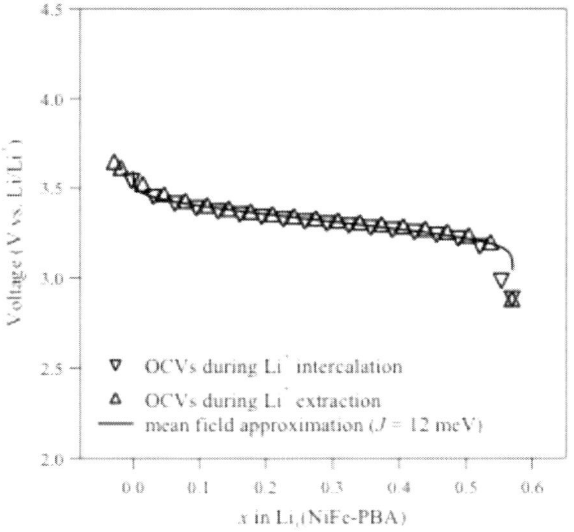

Figure 4. Open circuit voltages (OCVs) during Li^+ intercalation/extraction in Li_x(NiFe-PBA). The fitted curve with eq. (9) is also plotted.

As a typical PBA showing the reaction type (iii), $K_{0.2}Ni^{II}[Fe^{II}(CN)_6]_{0.1}[Fe^{III}(CN)_6]_{0.6}\cdot\square_{0.3}\cdot 4.7H_2O$ (hereafter denoted as NiFe-PBA) is obtained by adding Ni^{II} to $K_3[Fe^{III}(CN)_6]$ aqueous solution. The precise composition can be determined by combining both the elemental analysis (C, H, N, K, Ni and Fe) and Mössbauer spectroscopy. The open circuit voltages (OCVs) of Li_x(NiFe-PBA) in 1M $LiClO_4$/ethylene carbonate-diethyl carbonate (EC-DEC, 1:1 V/V%) electrolytes were recorded by the galvanostatic intermittent titration technique (GITT), and are shown in Figure 4 [21]. NiFe-PBA showed $0.6Li^+$ intercalation/extraction reversibly. Both the

Mössbauer spectra and magnetic properties confirmed the electrochemical reaction as:

$$0.6A^+ + e^- + K_{0.2}Ni^{II}[Fe^{II}(CN)_6]_{0.1}[Fe^{III}(CN)_6]_{0.6}\cdot\square_{0.3}\cdot 4.7H_2O$$

$$\leftrightarrow A_{0.6}K_{0.2}Ni^{II}[Fe^{II}(CN)_6]_{0.7}\cdot\square_{0.3}\cdot 4.7H_2O\ (A^+ = Li^+, Na^+ \text{ and } K^+).$$

Since the oxidation potential of Ni^{II} is too high, only the redox of Fe is available. The *ex-situ* X-ray diffraction patterns showed the gradual shift of the diffraction peak during ion intercalation/extraction, and no new peak emerged, thus A_x(NiFe-PBA) is the solid solution system for $0 < x < 0.6$. The OCVs for Li_x(NiFe-PBA) are well fitted with the eq. (9) (Figure 4). The interaction energy J is 12 meV/mol, which suggests weak repulsion between neighboring Li^+. The agreement between the experimental and mean field approximated OCVs supports the solid solution state, *i.e.*, random distribution of Li^+ in the host lattice of NiFe-PBA.

2.4. Charge Transfer at Interface

Charge transfer at the electrode-electrolyte interface plays an important role in the solid state electrochemistry, because ionic diffusion (in the solid solution system) or boundary migration (in the two phase system) occurs subsequent to the interfacial charge transfer.

Interfacial charge transfer during ion intercalation involves partial desolvation of ion, adsorption onto the electrode surface, surface diffusion at the electrode surface, and jump into the inside of the electrode. The energy barrier as a whole is regarded as the activation energy E_A for the interfacial charge transfer, which is one of the most fundamental criteria to evaluate the interface.

The electrochemical impedance spectroscopy (EIS) is a powerful technique to obtain E_A. The Nyquist plot from the EIS generally shows a semi-circle component corresponding to a RC circuit (an interfacial charge transfer resistance R_{CT} in parallel with an interfacial double layer capacitance). The temperature dependence of R_{CT} can provide E_A, which sheds light on the microscopic understanding of the interfacial charge transfer.

E_A for interfacial Li-ion transfer was intensively studied by T. Abe. For example, E_A at the interface between 1M $LiClO_4$/PC and *c*-axis oriented

Li_xCoO_2 thin film is 46 kJ/mol [31], while that at the interface between 1M $LiClO_4$/PC and $Li_xMn_2O_4$ is 54 kJ/mol [32].

As shown in Table 1, the temperature dependent EIS for the NiFe-PBA thin film electrode revealed that E_A at the interface between 1M $LiClO_4$/PC and NiFe-PBA is 61 kJ/mol, which is slightly larger than those for Li_xCoO_2 and $Li_xMn_2O_4$. Larger E_A should limit the rate of ion intercalation/extraction in the NiFe-PBA electrode.

The solvent effect on E_A is significant, since the interfacial charge transfer involves desolvation process. E_A at the interface between 1M $LiNO_3/H_2O$ and NiFe-PBA is 26 kJ/mol, which is much smaller than that with the PC electrolyte. Furthermore, E_A for the interfacial Na^+ transfer also decreases from 43 kJ/mol (PC) to 5 kJ/mol (H_2O).

Table 1. The activation energy for interfacial charge transfer between NiFe-PBA and various electrolytes

electrolyte	E_A (kJ/mol)
1 M $LiClO_4$/PC	61
1 M $NaClO_4$/PC	43
1 M $Mg(ClO_4)_2$/PC	No charge transfer
1 M $LiNO_3$(aq)	26
1 M $NaNO_3$(aq)	5
1 M $Mg(NO_3)_2$(aq)	27

The radii of hydrated Li^+ (2.37 Å) and Na^+ (1.83 Å) are slightly larger than the intercell bottleneck radius of PBAs (1.6 Å), thus charge transfer occurs after partial dehydration, while PC should be completely desolvated before charge transfer. The coordinated H_2O reduces the Coulombic repulsion between the ion and host, thus E_A is decreased. The fast kinetics by the hydration effect is effective to apply PBAs to the aqueous batteries (Section 3.2).

3. Application of PBA Electrodes for Rechargeable Batteries

3.1. Intercalation Electrodes for Rechargeable Batteries

The concept of a rocking chair battery, in which both anode and cathode materials are intercalation compounds, is effective to realize the high power and long cycle life of rechargeable batteries, because the structure of the host materials does not change drastically during the charge/discharge process. In this context, a variety of chalcogenides, graphite, oxides and polyanionic compounds has been reported as intercalation compounds.

A family of chalcogenides includes Li_xTiS_2, the first electrochemical Li^+ intercalation compound discovered in 1976 [17]. Li_xTiS_2 shows highly reversible Li^+ intercalation/extraction at about 2 V vs. Li/Li^+ via the solid solution process for $0 < x < 1$, which corresponds to the theoretical capacity of 239 mAh/g. Furthermore, the layered TiS_2 host can accommodate various other ions like Na^+ [33] and Mg^{2+} [34]. Other typical chalcogenides are layered metal selenides such as VSe_2 [35], chain compounds such as TiS_3 [36], and Chevrel compounds such as Mo_6Se_8 [20].

Graphite shows intercalation of various ions, and reversible Li^+ intercalation/extraction is used as an anodic reaction in the commercial Li-ion batteries. The theoretical capacity is 372 mAh/g, if the electrochemical reaction of

$$Li^+ + e^- + C_6 \leftrightarrow LiC_6,$$

is assumed. Since the ion intercalation into graphite frequently accompanies the co-intercalation of solvent molecules, the importance of solid-electrolyte interface (SEI) formation was emphasized by Z. Ogumi [37,38].

If the graphite anode is used, the concept of the rocking chair battery requires the cathode material containing the mobile ion, because a charge-discharge cycle should start from the charging process (ion extraction from the cathode and ion intercalation into the anode).

Therefore, various oxides containing Li were synthesized for the cathode materials of Li-ion batteries [39]. In particular, layered $LiCoO_2$ [40] and spinel $LiMn_2O_4$ [41], reported by J. B. Goodenough in 1980 and 1984, are used in the commercial Li-ion batteries, and show reversible electrochemical Li^+ intercalation/extraction as,

$LiCoO_2 \leftrightarrow xLi^+ + xe^- + Li_{1-x}CoO_2$,

and

$LiMn_2O_4 \leftrightarrow xLi^+ + xe^- + Li_{1-x}Mn_2O_4$.

The theoretical capacity for $0 < x < 1$ is 276 mAh/g for $LiCoO_2$ and 296 mAh/g for $LiMn_2O_4$, although the practical cutoff voltage reduces the accessible capacity. Other typical oxides are layered oxides such as $LiNiO_2$ [42], tunnel structure oxides such as α-MnO_2 (hollandite) [43], and amorphous oxides such as a-V_2O_5 [44].

$LiFePO_4$, another commercially used cathode material containing Li, was also proposed by J. B. Goodenough in 1997 [45]. As mentioned in section 2.2, $LiFePO_4$ shows reversible Li^+ intercalation/extraction via two phase process as,

$LiFePO_4 \leftrightarrow Li^+ + e^- + FePO_4$.

The theoretical capacity is 169 mAh/g, which is almost fully available in contrast to the oxides. Other polyanion compounds which show reversible ion intercalation have been reported by many groups. Li_2FeSiO_4 [46], $LiFeBO_3$ [47], and $Li_2FeP_2O_7$ [48] are typical examples.

Various oxides and polyanion compounds have been studied intensively: however, the study on a new class of electrode materials that provide reversible ion intercalation/extraction is of primary importance, because the strong industrial demands for low-cost, high energy, high power, and safe batteries. Recent progresses in application of PBA electrodes to rechargeable batteries are reviewed in the next section.

3.2. PBA Electrodes for Rechargeable Batteries

Application of PBAs to the electrode material of Li-ion batteries was first reported by N. Imanishi in 1999 [49,50]. PB delivered the reversible capacity of 110 mAh/g at the averaged voltage of about 3.0 V vs. Li/Li^+, while VFe-, MnFe-, CoFe-, NiFe-, and CuFe-PBA showed the reversible capacity of 65, 45, 70, 80 and 140 mAh/g, respectively. However, the available capacity is much smaller than that of $LiCoO_2$ and $LiFePO_4$, and the cycle stability was poor, thus the further studies were not carried out.

In 2010, M. Okubo re-evaluated the electrode performance of PBAs, and concluded that $K_{0.1}Mn^{II}[Fe^{III}(CN)_6]_{0.7}\cdot\square_{0.3}\cdot 4.3H_2O$ (MnFe-PBA) shows the reversible capacity of 60 mAh/g with high durability against the charge/discharge cycles (Figure 5) [8]. The detailed *ex-situ* XRD experiments revealed that the electrochemical reaction of $0.6Li^+$ $0.6e^-$ + MnFe-PBA $\leftrightarrow$ $Li_{0.6}$(MnFe-PBA) occurs via the solid solution state, and the corresponding change of the unit cell volume is only 3.5%. Soft x-ray absorption spectra for Fe and Mn *L*-edges clarified that C-coordinated Fe is redox-active while N-coordinated Mn is not redox-active on charge/discharge, which causes the low capacity of MnFe-PBA [9].

The electrochemical reaction of MnFe-PBA is classified into the reaction type (iii) (section 2.3), and the theoretical capacity is only 66 mAh/g. This result suggests that both C- and N-coordinated metal sites should be redox-active to increase the capacity.

$K_{0.1}Cu^{II}[Fe^{III}(CN)_6]_{0.7}\cdot\square_{0.3}\cdot 3.6H_2O$ (CuFe-PBA) has the redox-active N-coordinated Cu due to the accessible Cu^{II}/Cu^{I} redox couple.

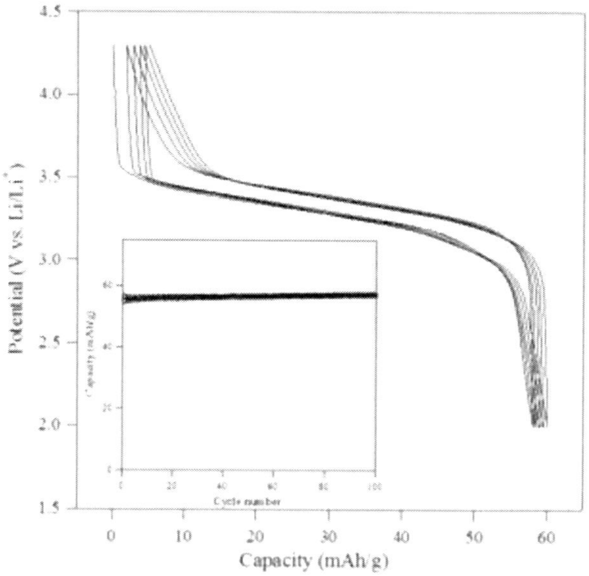

Figure 5. The charge-discharge curves at the specific current of 50 mA/g for the MnFe-PBA electrode. The cutoff voltage is 4.3 and 2.0 V vs. Li/Li$^+$, and the electrolyte is 1M $LiClO_4$/EC-DEC. The inset shows the cycle stability during 100 cycles.

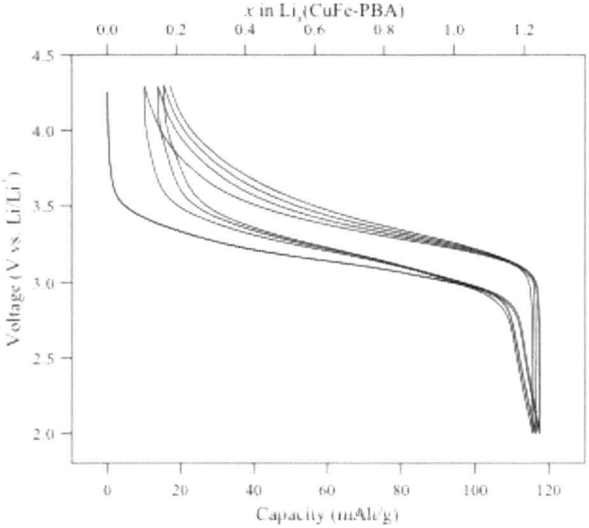

Figure 6. The charge-discharge curves at the specific current of 30 mA/g for the CuFe-PBA electrode. The cutoff voltage is 4.3 and 2.0 V vs. Li/Li^+, and the electrolyte is 1M $LiClO_4$/EC-DEC.

The charge/discharge experiments revealed that CuFe-PBA shows an exceptional reaction as,

$$1.2Li^+ + 1.2e^- + K_{0.1}Cu^{II}[Fe^{III}(CN)_6]_{0.7}\cdot\square_{0.3}\cdot 3.6H_2O$$

$$\leftrightarrow Li_{1.2}K_{0.1}Cu^{II}{}_{0.5}Cu^{I}{}_{0.5}[Fe^{II}(CN)_6]_{0.7}\cdot\square_{0.3}\cdot 3.6H_2O,$$

where both Fe and Cu is redox-active. As shown in Figure 6, the reversible capacity is increased to 120 mAh/g [51], but is still smaller than that of the oxides. In addition, the cycle stability is extremely low, because Li^+ intercalation gives rise to formation of an unstable phase at the surface.

The causes for the small capacity of PBAs with the vacancy are as follows.

(a) The vacancy in PBAs decreases the amount of redox-active C-coordinated sites.
(b) The weight of water in the vacancy increases the molar mass of the host.
(c) The reaction types (iii) and (iv) (section 2.3) cannot provide the two-electron reaction except CuFe-PBA

Therefore, in order to enhance the reversible capacity, the reaction type (i) for PBAs without the vacancy is needed, because the theoretical capacity of $2Li^+ + 2e^- + M^{III}[M^{III}(CN)_6] \leftrightarrow Li_2M^{II}[M^{II}(CN)_6]$ exceeds 200 mAh/g.

In this context, a vacancy-suppressed MnMn-PBA electrode was investigated. $K_2Mn^{II}[Mn^{II}(CN)_6]$, which is synthesized by mixing KCN and Mn^{II} in aqueous solution, has been studied from the viewpoint of magnetism since 1968 [5,52]. This material is known to contain only less than 0.3 wt% of H, implying that it has few vacancies and little zeolitic water. The elemental analysis for the synthesized compound suggested the precise composition of $K_{1.72}Mn^{II}[Mn^{II}(CN)_6]_{0.93}\cdot\square_{0.07}\cdot 0.65H_2O$, however, the amount of the vacancy (7%) is largely suppressed compared with that in MnFe-PBA and CuFe-PBA (30%). The electrochemical K^+ extraction was carried out to obtain the vacancy-suppressed $Mn[Mn(CN)_6]_{0.93}\cdot\square_{0.07}\cdot 0.65H_2O$ (MnMn-PBA), which was then tested as the electrode material of the Li-ion battery. The charge/discharge experiments showed that the reversible capacity of MnMn-PBA is 200 mAh/g at the averaged potential of 3.1 V vs. Li/Li^+ (Figure 7) [53]. The OCVs in Figure 7 show two plateaus at 3.7 and 3.0 V, which suggests that both C-coordinated and N-coordinated Mn sites are redox-active.

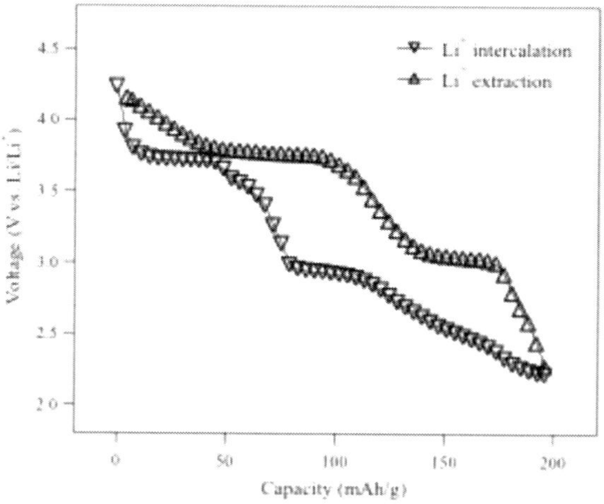

Figure 7. The open circuit voltages for vacancy-suppressed MnMn-PBA.

The available capacity almost agrees with the theoretical capacity of the reaction type (i), which is larger than that of $LiCoO_2$ and $LiFePO_4$. Although the poor cycle stability of vacancy-suppressed MnMn-PBA needs further optimization, the enhanced capacity opened new perspectives in application to batteries.

Application of PBAs to aqueous batteries was proposed by Y. Cui [54-56]. The aqueous batteries use inexpensive aqueous electrolytes, which is suitable for the grid scale energy storage system. As mentioned in section 2.4, the hydrated ions can be intercalated into PBAs with a small E_A due to the screening effect of hydration, thus NiFe- and CuFe-PBA allow retention of 66% of the initial capacity at a very high charge/discharge rate (41.7 C for NiFe-PBA and 83 C for CuFe-PBA) and the long cycle life over 5000 cycles. Unfortunately, the precise composition of PBAs was not determined in these reports, and the detailed analysis of the reaction has not been carried out, but CuFe-PBA did not have instability of CuFe-PBA which was observed with the organic electrolytes. These results clearly emphasize the importance of the electrolyte.

The Na-ion battery with the PBA electrodes was also proposed by J. B. Goodenough [57]. Although the precise composition and detailed electrochemical reaction were not clarified, PB, MnFe-, NiFe-, CuFe-, CoFe- and ZnFe-PBAs showed reversible Na^+ intercalation/extraction with the organic electrolyte (PC). The highest capacity is 100 mAh/g for PB, and this result suggests that PBAs is applicable to the electrode materials of the Na-ion battery.

CONCLUSION

Since the discovery by Prof. Itaya, the electrochemical properties of PBAs have been investigated from the viewpoint of electrochromism. However, in the 2010s, the strong industrial demands for low cost, high power, higher energy and safe batteries are focusing application of PBAs to the electrode materials of batteries. MnFe-PBA is highly durable against the charge-discharge processes over 100 cycles, while vacancy-suppressed MnMn-PBA can show the reversible capacity of *ca.* 200 mAh/g, which exceeds that of conventional cathode materials. Furthermore, some groups have proposed post Li-ion batteries such as aqueous batteries or Na-ion batteries with the PBA electrodes.

The main drawbacks of the PBA electrodes are, for example, zeolitic water and theoretical capacity in the unit of Ah/L. Zeolitic water involved in PBAs with the vacancy could contaminate the organic electrolyte, which seriously degrades the anode materials. The theoretical capacity in the unit of

Ah/L is the other important criterion of the cathode materials, because larger theoretical capacity gives smaller batteries. For example, the theoretical capacity of MnMn-PBA is 267 Ah/L, while that of $LiCoO_2$ is 699 Ah/L. The other important issue is the safety issue. The cyanides in the batteries must be secure during the long cycle life.

ACKNOWLEDGMENTS

It is a great pleasure to acknowledge the followings for their significant contributions to this work: T. Kudo, I. Honma, N. Kojima, T. Mizokawa, Y. Mizuno, D. Asakura, E. Hosono, Y. Ohno, and Y. Nanba.

REFERENCES

[1] M. Verdaguer, G. S. Girolami, Magnetic Prussian blue analogs, in Magnetism: Molecules to Materials V, Wiley-VCH, Weinheim, 2005.

[2] A. Ludi, H. U. Gudel, *Inorg. Chem.*, (1970) 9, 2224.

[3] J. H. Buser, A. Ludi, H. U. Gudel, *J. Chem. Soc., Chem. Commun.*, (1972) 1299.

[4] E. Fluck, W. Kerler, W. Neuwirth, *Angew. Chem. Int. Ed.,* (1963) 2, 277.

[5] J. H. Her, P. W. Stephens, C. M. Kareis, J. G. Moore, K. S. Min, J. W. Park, G. Bali, B. S. Kennon, J. S. Miller, *Inorg. Chem.*, (2010) 49, 1524.

[6] C. M. Kareis, S. H. Lapidus, J. H. Her, P. W. Stephens, J. S. Miller, *J. Am. Chem. Soc.*, (2012) 134, 2246.

[7] S. Margadonna, K. Prassides, A. N. Fitch, *J. Am. Chem. Soc.*, (2004) 126, 15390.

[8] M. Okubo, D. Asakura, Y. Mizuno, J. D. Kim, T. Mizokawa, T. Kudo, I. Honma, *J. Phys. Chem. Lett.*, (2010) 1, 2063.

[9] D. Asakura, M. Okubo, Y. Mizuno, T. Kudo, H. S. Zhou, K. Amemiya, F. M. F. de Groot, J. L. Chen, W. C. Wang, P. A. Glans, C. Chang, J. Guo, I. Honma, *Phys. Rev. B*, (2011) 84, 045117.

[10] M. B. Robin, *Inorg. Chem.*, (1962) 1, 337.

[11] S. Ferlay, T. Mallah, R. Ouahes, P. Veillet, M. Verdaguer, *Nature*, (1995) 378, 701.

[12] O. Sato, T. Iyoda, A. Fujishima, K. Hashimoto, *Science*, (1996) 272, 704.
[13] M. Verdaguer, A. Bluezen, V. Marvaud, J. Vaissermann, M. Seuleiman, C. Desplanches, A. Scuiller, C. Train, R. Garde, G. Gelly, C. Lomenech, I. Rosenman, P. Veillet, C. Cartier, F. Villain, *Coord. Chem. Rev.*, (1999) 192, 1023.
[14] S. Ohkoshi, H. Tokoro, K. Hashimoto, *Coord. Chem. Rev.*, (2005) 249, 1830.
[15] M. Faraday, Philosophical transactions of the royal society of London, Richard and John Taylor, London, 1838.
[16] P. G. Bruce, ed., Solid state electrochemistry, Cambridge University Press, Cambridge, 1995.
[17] M. S. Whittingham, *Science*, (1976) 192, 1126.
[18] A. Yoshino, *Angew. Chem. Int. Ed.*, (2012) 51, 5798.
[19] V. D. Neff, *J. Electrochem. Soc.*, (1978) 125, 886.
[20] S. T. Coleman, W. R. McKinnon, J. R. Dahn, *Phys. Rev. B*, (1984) 29, 4147.
[21] Y. Mizuno, M. Okubo, K. Kagesawa, D. Asakura, T. Kudo, H. S. Zhou, K. Oh-ishi, A. Okazawa, N. Kojima, *Inorg. Chem.*, (2012) 51, 10311.
[22] A. Yamada, S. C. Chung, K. Hinokuma, *J. Electrochem. Soc.*, (2001) 148, A224.
[23] A. Yamada, H. Koizumi, S. Nishimura, N. Sonoyama, R. Kanno, M. Yonemura, T. Nakamura, Y. Kobayashi, *Nat. Mat.*, (2006) 5, 357.
[24] M. Tang, H. Y. Huang, N. Meethong, Y. H. Kao, W. C. Carter, Y. M. Chiang, *Chem. Mater.*, (2009) 21, 1557.
[25] R. Malik, F. Zhou, G. Ceder, *Nat. Mat.*, (2011) 10, 587.
[26] G. K. Singh, G. Ceder, M. Z. Bazant, *Electrochim. Acta*, (2008) 53, 7599.
[27] M. Wagemaker, A. P. M. Kentgens, F. M. Mulder, *Nature*, (2002) 418, 397.
[28] M. Wagemaker, D. P. Singh, W. J. H. Borghols, U. Lafont, L. Haverkate, V. K. Peterson, F. M. Mulder, *J. Am. Chem. Soc.*, (2011) 133, 10222.
[29] K. Itaya, I. Uchida, *Acc. Chem. Res.*, (1986) 19, 162.
[30] T. Ozeki, I. Watanabe, S. Ikeda, *J. Electroanal. Chem.*, (1987) 236, 209.
[31] I. Yamada, Y. Iriyama, T. Abe, Z. Ogumi, *J. Power Sources*, (2007) 172, 933.
[32] S. Kobayashi, Y. Uchimoto, *J. Phys. Chem. B*, (2005) 109, 13322.
[33] B. M. L. Rao, *J. Electrochem. Soc.*, (1978) 125, C471.

[34] P. G. Bruce, F. Krok, P. Lightfoot, J. L. Nowinski, V. C. Gibson, *Solid State Ionics*, (1992) 53, 351.
[35] M. S. Whittingham, *Mat. Res. Bull.*, (1978) 13, 959.
[36] M. Zanini, J. L. Shaw, G. J. Tennenhouse, *J. Electrochem. Soc.*, (1981) 128, 1647.
[37] S. K. Jeong, M. Inaba, Y. Iriyama, T. Abe, Z. Ogumi, *Electrochim. Acta*, (2002) 47, 1975.
[38] Z. Ogumi, T. Abe, T. Fukutsuka, S. Yamate, Y. Iriyama, *J. Power Sources*, (2004) 127, 72.
[39] G. A. Nazri, G. Pistoia, *ed.*, *Lithium Batteries: Science and Technology*, Springer, 2008.
[40] K. Mizushima, P. C. Jones, P. J. Wiseman, J. B. Goodenough, *Mat. Res. Bull.*, (1980) 15, 783.
[41] M. M. Thackeray, P. J. Johnson, L. A. Depicciotto, P. G. Bruce, J. B. Goodenough, *Mat. Res. Bull.*, (1984) 19, 179.
[42] J. R. Dahn, U. Vonsacken, M. W. Juzkow, H. Aljanaby, *J. Electrochem. Soc.*, (1991) 138, 2207.
[43] S. Bach, J. P. Pereiraramos, N. Baffier, *Solid State Ionics*, (1995) 80, 151.
[44] Y. Sakurai, J. Yamaki, *J. Electrochem. Soc.*, (1988) 135, 791.
[45] A. K. Padhi, K. S. Nanjundaswamy, J. B. Goodenough, *J. Electrochem. Soc.*, (1997) 144, 1188.
[46] A. Nyten, A. Abouimrane, M. Armand, T. Gustafsson, J. O. Thomas, *Electrochem. Commun.*, (2005) 7, 156.
[47] V. Legagneur, Y. An, A. Mosbah, R. Portal, A. Le gal La Salle, A. Verbaere, D. Guyomard, Y. Piffard, *Solid State Ionics*, (2001) 139, 37.
[48] S. Nishimura, M. Nakamura, R. Natsui, A. Yamada, *J. Am. Chem. Soc.*, (2010) 132, 13596.
[49] N. Imanishi, T. Morikawa, J. Kondo, Y. Takeda, O. Yamamoto, N. Kinugasa, T. Yamagishi, *J. Power Sources*, (1999) 79, 215.
[50] N. Imanishi, T. Morikawa, J. Kondo, R. Yamane, Y. Takeda, O. Yamamoto, H. Sakaebe, M. Tabuchi, *J. Power Sources*, (1999) 81-82, 530.
[51] M. Okubo, D. Asakura, Y. Mizuno, T. Kudo, H. S. Zhou, A. Okazawa, N. Kojima, K. Ikedo, T. Mizokawa, I. Honma, *Angew. Chem. Int. Ed.*, (2011) 50, 6269.
[52] A. M. Qureshi, A. G. Sharpe, *J. Inorg. Nucl. Chem.*, (1968) 30, 2269.

[53] D. Asakura, M. Okubo, Y. Mizuno, T. Kudo, H. S. Zhou, K. Ikedo, T. Mizokawa, A. Okazawa, N. Kojima, *J. Phys. Chem. C*, (2012) 116, 8364.

[54] C. D. Wessells, R. A. Huggins, Y. Cui, *Nat. Commun.*, (2011) 2, 550.

[55] C. D. Wessells, S. V. Peddada, R. A. Huggins, Y. Cui, *Nano Lett.*, (2011) 11, 5421.

[56] C. D. Wessells, S. V. Peddada, M. T. McDowell, R. A. Huggins, Y. Cui, *J. Electrochem. Soc.*, (2012) 159, A98.

[57] Y. Lu, L. Wang, J. Cheng, J. B. Goodenough, *Chem. Commun.*, (2012) 48, 6544.

INDEX

A

absorption spectra, 102
abstraction, 17
acetylcholine, 27, 33
acid, 6, 10, 13, 16, 21, 24, 25, 26, 27, 33, 36, 41, 44, 45, 52
acidic, 15, 53
acidosis, 28
activation energy, 98, 99
acute poisoning, viii, 23
adenine, 12, 19
adjustment, 67
adsorption, viii, 1, 9, 14, 15, 98
adverse effects, 39
aetiology, 37
aggregation, 4
alanine, 6
aldehydes, 10, 12, 25
algae, 41
algorithm, 74, 75
amblyopia, 31, 38
amines, 17
amino, 41, 45
amino acid(s), viii, 2, 6, 7, 9, 10, 12, 16, 17, 20, 27, 29, 33, 37
ammonia, vii, 9, 10, 12, 24
ammonium, 16, 18
angstroms, 71, 72
anoxia, viii, 23, 27
antagonism, 45
antioxidant, 35
apoptosis, 40
aqueous solutions, 10, 11, 18, 20, 74
arginine, 7
arthropods, 6, 18
aspartate, 27, 33, 38, 45
assessment, 35, 65
asteroids, 5
ataxia, 32, 34
atmosphere, 3, 8, 11, 17, 19, 21
atoms, 12, 88, 89
atrophy, 31, 34, 41
axons, 32

B

bacteria, 6, 18, 26, 37, 40
batteries, vii, ix, 87, 91, 95, 99, 100, 101, 105, 106
behaviors, 11
biochemistry, 13, 20
birds, 30, 38
biuret, 7
blood, 28, 31
body weight, 27, 29, 34
Boltzmann constant, 92
bonding, 52
bone, 39
brain, 28, 36, 39, 42, 44
breakdown, 25, 36
building blocks, 7, 10

C

cadmium, 52
calcium, 15, 27, 30, 33, 35, 45
cancer, 24, 40
capsule, 34
carbohydrates, 25
carbon, vii, 24
carbon dioxide (CO2), 12, 16
carbon monoxide, 12
carboxylic acid(s), viii, 2, 7, 10, 12, 16, 17, 20, 26, 33, 36
catalysis, 13
catalytic activity, 5
cathode materials, 91, 100, 105, 106
cation, 49, 52, 88, 90
cattle, 27, 32, 40
cell differentiation, 29
cellular hypoxia, viii, 23
central nervous system, 27, 32
central nervous system (CNS), 27, 30, 32, 33
cerebellum, 32
CFI, 41
chalcogenides, 100
chemical, vii, viii, ix, 1, 2, 3, 4, 5, 6, 7, 8, 9, 10, 11, 13, 14, 15, 16, 17, 18, 20, 23, 24, 42, 44, 48, 58, 60, 61, 88, 91, 92, 93
chemical bonds, 11
chemical interaction, ix, 15, 48
chemical properties, 6
chemical reactions, vii, 1, 3, 4, 11, 14
cigarette smoking, 24
classification, 53, 88
clay minerals, 5, 15, 20, 21
C-N, 17
coma, 19
commercial, 100
community, 38
competition, 11
compilation, 58
composition, 76, 88, 89, 92, 96, 97, 104, 105
compounds, vii, 1, 2, 8, 9, 10, 11, 12, 17, 18, 24, 42, 90, 91, 100, 101
conduction, ix, 87, 91
conductivity, 90
conductor, 91
configuration, 67, 92, 93
conjugation, 26, 33
consumption, 31, 34, 39, 41
convection model, 66
coordination, vii, ix, 87, 88
copper, ix, 37, 48, 52, 56, 58, 76, 81
correlation(s), 31, 48, 64, 65, 66, 67, 68, 69, 72, 76, 78, 80
cortex, 32
cosmetic, 50
cosmic rays, 3, 4, 5
cost, 101, 105
cotyledon, 34
crops, 34
crust, 4, 5
crystal structure, 88
crystals, 30
CV, 95, 96, 97
cyanamide, 18
cyanide, vii, viii, ix, 6, 8, 11, 18, 19, 20, 23, 24, 25, 26, 27, 28, 29, 30, 31, 32, 33, 34, 35, 36, 37, 38, 39, 40, 41, 42, 43, 44, 45, 47, 50, 51, 52, 53, 54, 55, 56, 57, 58, 61, 62, 66, 74, 75, 76, 77, 80, 81, 82, 83, 84, 87, 88, 89, 90, 91
cyanide poisoning, viii, 23, 24, 28, 30, 35, 37, 39, 42, 43
cyanocobalamin, 26
cyanosis, 51
cycles, 33, 102, 105
cyclooxygenase, 38
cysteine, 26, 33
cytochrome, viii, 23, 27, 33
cytotoxic anoxia, viii, 23

D

database, 40
deaths, 38, 41
decay, 3, 4
decomposition, 11, 16, 17
defects, 34

deficiency, 30, 37
degradation, 16, 84
dehydration, 99
dementia, 31
demyelination, 32
deposition, 4, 29
deposits, 5
derivatives, vii, 1, 7, 8, 20
desorption, 66
detection, 7, 20
detoxification, viii, 23, 27, 35, 41
diabetes, 28, 30, 31, 37, 40, 42, 45
diet, 24, 31, 38, 39, 41, 42
diffraction, 98
diffusion, ix, 48, 50, 63, 65, 68, 71, 72, 73, 83, 87, 91, 98
diffusion process, 68
discharges, 8
diseases, 31
disorder, 32
dissociation, viii, 47, 49, 52, 77
distribution, 4, 5, 35, 52, 53, 57, 78, 98
DNA, 3
dogs, 28, 29, 31, 39, 41
dopamine, 27, 33, 36
dosing, 43, 44
drugs, viii, 23, 24
drying, 25, 42
durability, 102
dynamic systems, 60, 75
dyspnea, 28

E

editors, 35, 37, 39, 41, 42
effluents, 24
EIS, 98, 99
electric charge, 95
electric current, 91
electrochemical impedance, 98
electrochemistry, ix, 87, 90, 91, 93, 95, 96, 98, 107
electrochromism, ix, 87, 105
electrode surface, 98
electrodes, vii, ix, 87, 90, 91, 101, 105
electrolyte, 90, 98, 99, 100, 102, 103, 105
electron(s), ix, 10, 11, 27, 87, 88, 90, 103
electronic structure, 89
electroplating, vii, viii, 23, 24, 50
endocrine, 39
energy, viii, 1, 3, 4, 5, 8, 9, 10, 11, 13, 14, 16, 20, 48, 72, 93, 95, 98, 101, 105
entropy, 92, 93, 95
environment(s), viii, 2, 4, 5, 8, 9, 13, 14, 17, 23
enzymatic combination, viii, 23
enzyme(s), viii, 6, 23, 25, 26, 27, 30, 31, 33, 41, 44
epithelial cells, 28
equilibrium, ix, 48, 50, 51, 53, 54, 55, 58, 60, 61, 62, 63
equipment, ix, 47, 48, 49, 50, 51, 61, 62, 64, 65, 66, 73, 74, 75, 80
ethylene, 97
etiology, 31, 44
evidence, 40, 42, 44
evolution, vii, 1, 2, 3, 5, 6, 7, 8, 9, 10, 16, 17, 18, 20, 21, 75
excitation, 10, 16, 36
excretion, 30
execution, 24
exposure, viii, 23, 24, 28, 29, 31, 34, 37, 41, 43, 44, 45, 51, 79
extraction, ix, 24, 87, 90, 91, 92, 93, 95, 97, 98, 99, 100, 101, 104, 105
extracts, 24

F

FAS, 34
fat, 29
fiber(s), 49, 67, 68, 69
fibrosis, 31
fires, vii, 24, 38
fixation, 5
fluid, 40
follicles, 30
food, 26, 38, 39
force, 50, 62, 63
formamide, 19

formation, vii, 1, 2, 5, 7, 8, 9, 10, 12, 17, 27, 33, 34, 93, 100, 103
formula, 88
free energy, 91
free radicals, 4, 9, 27, 32
freezing, 9, 25
fruits, 6, 43
fuel cell, 91
fungi, 6

G

GABA, 27, 33
gamma rays, 5
gas sensors, 51
gastrointestinal tract, 26
genus, 25, 30
geometry, ix, 48, 61, 64, 65
gestation, 44
gland, 30
gluconeogenesis, 31
glucose, 31
glucose tolerance, 34
glutamate, 27, 33, 36, 40
glutamic acid, 6, 27, 33, 36
glutathione, 27, 33
glycine, 7
glycoside, 24, 31, 34
goiter, 38
graphite, 100
grass, 25
grazing, 32, 36, 40
growth, 28, 29, 39
growth hormone, 29, 39
guanine, 7

H

half-life, 4
hearing loss, 31
helium, 5
hemorrhage, 28, 31
hepatocytes, 28, 34
hepatotoxicity, 44
heterogeneity, 40
heterogeneous medium, vii, 1, 13
hippocampus, 32, 33
history, 4
Hmong, 38
homicide, 24
homovanillic acid, 36
hormone(s), 29, 30, 39
horses, 32, 34
host, ix, 87, 91, 92, 93, 94, 95, 98, 99, 100, 103
human, 34
human health, 51
hydrocarbons, 9
hydrogen cyanide (HCN), vii, viii, 1, 6, 7, 8, 9, 10, 12, 13, 14, 15, 16, 17, 18, 19, 21, 25, 26, 27, 38, 47, 49, 50, 51, 52, 53, 54, 57, 58, 59, 60, 61, 62, 63, 64, 65, 66, 68, 71, 72, 73, 74, 75, 76, 77, 78, 79, 80, 81, 82, 83
hydrolysis, viii, 2, 7, 9, 12, 13, 16, 17
hydrosphere, vii, 1
hydroxyl, 52
hyperglycemia, 28
hypotensive, 24
hypothesis, viii, 2, 29
hypothyroidism, 28, 29
hypoxia, viii, 23, 27, 33, 51

I

ideal, 63, 68, 93
identification, ix, 48
in vitro, 38, 40
in vivo, 38
incidence, 34, 45
incomplete combustion, 24
indirect effect, 11
individuals, 30
induction, 39
industries, viii, 47, 83
industry, 37, 50, 58, 75
ingestion, 25, 26, 34, 40, 43, 51
inhibition, 36, 40, 43
injury, 30, 31, 41

inositol, 36
insulin, 30
interface, 50, 58, 60, 61, 63, 65, 66, 78, 80, 98, 99, 100
interference, 42
intermediaries, 12
interstellar dust, 2
intervention, 9
intoxication, 24, 29, 33, 34, 35, 36, 37, 39, 41, 42, 43, 45
investment, ix, 48
iodine, 29, 38
ionization, 10
ionizing radiation, vii, 1, 3, 4, 5, 9, 10, 16, 17, 20
ions, 4, 11, 27, 33, 52, 91, 92, 93, 100, 105
iron, 27
irradiation, 4, 8, 11, 12, 14, 16, 18, 19, 90

K

K^+, 31, 88, 90, 96, 98, 104
ketones, 12, 25
kidney, 41
kinetics, 11, 43, 60, 95, 99

L

lactation, 43
lactic acid, 35
lakes, 4
laminar, 65, 67
L-arginine, 45
leaching, 75, 85
lead, 10, 82
leaks, 79
lesions, 28, 30, 31, 32, 34, 36, 41, 44
ligand, 90
light, 90, 98
lipid metabolism, 29
lipid peroxidation, 27, 32, 35, 41
lipids, 39
liquid phase, ix, 10, 48, 49, 50, 58, 60, 61, 62, 63, 65, 68, 73, 74, 75, 78, 79, 80, 83
liquids, 73
liver, viii, 23
livestock, 41
low temperatures, viii, 2, 58
lumen, 67

M

magnesium, 15
magnetic properties, 90, 98
magnetism, 104
magnetization, 90
magnitude, 61, 73, 83
malnutrition, 34, 37, 40
manufacturing, vii, 24
mass, viii, 48, 49, 51, 54, 60, 61, 62, 63, 64, 65, 66, 67, 68, 69, 73, 74, 75, 76, 78, 80, 81, 83, 95, 103
materials, vii, ix, 10, 16, 87, 100, 101, 105
matter, 4, 5, 17, 32
measurements, 19, 83
medical, 37
medulla oblongata, 32
melatonin, 45
mellitus, 39
melting, 6
membranes, 28, 33, 66, 67, 69
mesencephalon, 32
metabolic, 43
metabolism, 18, 19, 25, 27, 28, 29, 36, 37, 38, 39, 40, 45
metabolites, 44
metals, 27, 51, 52, 56, 77, 90
meteorites, 2, 7, 16
methodology, 83
Mexico, 1
Mg^{2+}, 100
mice, 32, 35, 39
microenvironments, 5
midbrain, 32
migration, 98
miscarriage, 34
mixing, 88, 92, 93, 104
models, 58, 59, 68, 72, 82
modifications, 83

modules, 67
molar volume, 73
molecular weight, 12, 71, 73
molecules, 2, 3, 5, 7, 8, 9, 10, 11, 13, 15
monomers, 10
morphology, 95
motor neuron disease, 44
mucous membranes, 26
multiplier, 93
muscle spasms, 28
mycotoxins, 41

N

Na^+, 15, 31, 88, 90, 91, 92, 98, 99, 100, 105
National Academy of Sciences, 20
necrosis, 31
nervous system, 27, 32
neuritis, 31, 37, 41
neurological disease, 41
neuronal cells, 35
neurons, 27, 32, 33, 41
neuropathy, 31, 37, 40, 41, 42
neurotoxicity, 33, 38, 45
neurotransmitters, 27, 33
nickel, ix, 48, 52, 56, 58, 76, 81
nitric oxide, 27, 33, 35, 38
nitric oxide synthase, 38
nitrogen, 8, 18
nitroprusside, viii, 23, 24, 37, 43
non-smokers, 45
nuclei, 5, 18, 32
nucleic acid, 10, 20
nutrition, 41

O

oceans, 4, 5
oligomers, 7, 12, 17
operations, viii, 47, 51, 73, 83, 85
optimization, 50, 105
organ, 31
organic compounds, viii, 2, 3, 4, 7, 10, 20
organic matter, 19
organism, viii, 23
organs, 34, 35
oxidation, 98
oxidative stress, 40
oxygen, 11, 13, 28, 39

P

paints, 88
pancreas, 31
pancreatitis, 35, 37, 41, 42
parallel, 78, 98
parenchyma, 30
paresis, 28
partition, 62
pastures, 34, 36
pathogens, 19
pathways, 6, 11
peptide(s), 7, 12
peptides, 7
perchlorate, 38
petechiae, 28
petroleum, 15
pH, viii, ix, 1, 7, 10, 11, 15, 45, 48, 51, 52, 53, 54, 56, 57, 66, 76, 77, 79, 81, 82
pharmacokinetics, 43
pheochromocytoma, 39
photolysis, 8, 19
physical properties, 51, 61, 65, 68, 74
pigs, 28, 29, 32, 40, 44
placenta, 34
planets, 2, 17
plants, viii, 6, 19, 23, 24, 25, 26, 30, 31, 34, 37, 39, 41, 42, 43
plasma levels, 29
pleasure, 106
poison, 44
polar, 9
pollution, 36
polyamides, 12, 17
polyesters, 12, 17
polymer(s), vii, ix, 8, 9, 12, 20, 87, 91
polymerization, 9
ponds, 4, 75
pons, 32

porosity, 15, 67, 68
potassium, 5, 27, 44
poverty, 41
predation, 25
pregnancy, 34
present value, 4
primordial epoch, viii, 1, 14
principles, 10
project, ix, 48, 51
promoter, 39
proportionality, 82
protection, 13
protein synthesis, 20
proteins, 10
protons, 5
Prussian blue analog (PBA), ix, 87, 88, 89, 90, 97, 98, 99, 100, 101, 102, 103, 104, 105, 106
psychosis, 31
purines, viii, 2, 17, 21
pyrolysis, 3

Q

quaternary ammonium, 16

R

radiation, 3, 4, 5, 7, 11, 20, 21
radiation chemistry, vii, 1, 10, 16, 17, 18
radical formation, 33
radicals, 11, 17, 27, 33
radio, 45
radioactive isotopes, 3
radioisotope, 37
radius, 73, 88, 90, 99
reactants, 13
reaction mechanism, 11
reactions, viii, 1, 2, 3, 4, 10, 11, 13, 14, 17, 25, 97
reactive oxygen, 38
reactivity, 9
reagents, 8
receptors, 29
recovery process(es), 51, 66, 80
red blood cells, 28
registry, 35
regulations, viii, 47, 50, 51, 78, 81, 83
relevance, vii, 1
remediation, viii, 47
repulsion, 98, 99
resistance, ix, 6, 26, 48, 62, 63, 78, 80, 83, 98
respiration, 28
respiratory arrest, 28
respiratory rate, 28
response, 30
risk, viii, 38, 47, 51, 66, 81, 83
risk factors, 45
risks, 82
RNA, 3
rodents, 34
room temperature, 90

S

safety, viii, 47, 50, 83, 106
salts, 52
science, 90
secretion, 29
sediments, 5
seizure, 36
selenium, 30, 36, 37, 38
serum, 44
sheep, 27, 29, 30, 32, 35, 36, 38
showing, 6, 10, 95, 97
signs, 28
silver, vii, 24, 36, 50
simulation, 8, 74, 82
simulations, ix, 48
skin, 51
society, 107
sodium, 15, 24, 28, 36, 37, 43, 91
solid state, ix, 87, 90, 91, 95, 96, 97, 98
solid surfaces, 9, 13
solubility, 52, 95
solution, ix, 7, 10, 11, 13, 48, 51, 52, 53, 54, 56, 57, 58, 60, 61, 62, 66, 68, 74, 75, 76,

77, 78, 80, 82, 83, 88, 89, 92, 93, 95, 97, 98, 100, 102, 104
solvent molecules, 100
spastic, 32, 45
species, vii, viii, ix, 4, 11, 17, 23, 25, 26, 30, 31, 32, 38, 39, 48, 49, 52, 53, 54, 55, 56, 57, 72, 77, 83
spectroscopy, 88, 97, 98
spinal cord, 32
stability, 52, 53, 54, 101, 102, 103, 104
stars, 8
state(s), ix, 2, 4, 48, 74, 75, 90, 91, 92, 95, 96, 98, 102, 107
steel, vii, 24
stomach, 26
storage, ix, 16, 66, 85, 87, 105
stress, vii, 1
strong interaction, 93
structure, 8, 9, 15, 36, 88, 89, 100, 101
subcutaneous tissue, 29
suicide, 24, 38, 45
sulfate, 29
sulfur, viii, 23, 26, 29, 37, 41
supplier, 67
suppliers, 66
surface area, 34
surface tension, 95
swelling, 15, 21
syndrome, 41
synthesis, viii, 2, 3, 4, 6, 8, 9, 10, 13, 19, 21, 23, 30

T

tanks, 66, 69, 75, 76, 80
target, 74
techniques, 2, 11
technologies, 90
temperature, ix, 4, 7, 10, 48, 53, 54, 56, 58, 59, 68, 71, 72, 73, 90, 95, 98, 99
temperature dependence, 98
terrorism, 42
therapeutic use, 43
thermal energy, 3
thermodynamic equilibrium, ix, 48, 49
thermodynamics, 91, 95
thiosulphate, 43
thorium, 5
thyroid, viii, 23, 34, 38, 39, 40
thyroid gland, 29, 30, 35, 36, 45
tissue, 31, 32, 44, 51
tobacco, 31
toxic effect, viii, 23, 29, 33, 42
toxicity, vii, 6, 24, 25, 26, 27, 32, 34, 35, 39, 42, 43, 44
toxicology, 24, 29
trachea, 28
transactions, 107
transformation, 29, 33
transformation product, 33
transition metal, 88, 89
transport, ix, 27, 36, 48, 66
treatment, 24, 32, 40
triiodothyronine, 30
turbulence, 78, 80, 83

U

universal gas constant, 54
uranium, 5
urea, 12
UV irradiation, 21
UV light, 8
UV radiation, 3, 4, 7

V

vacancies, 104
valence, 90
validation, 64
velocity, 50, 65, 67, 68, 69
victims, 38
viscosity, 65, 68, 73
vitamin B1, 26, 38
vitamin B12, 26, 38
vitamin B12 deficiency, 38
volatilization, ix, 48, 60, 62, 63, 85

W

water, 6, 10, 11, 17, 18, 52, 68, 71, 72, 73, 74, 83, 88, 89, 103, 104, 105
weight gain, viii, 23, 29
white matter, 28, 32, 34
workers, 36, 37, 58, 82
workplace, 50
worldwide, 24

X

X-ray diffraction (XRD), 98, 102

Y

yield, 11

Z

zinc, ix, 48, 52